Handbook of Blood Gas/Acid-Base Interpretation

Ashfaq Hasan

Handbook of Blood Gas/ Acid-Base Interpretation

Second Edition

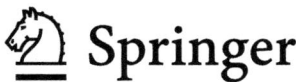 Springer

Ashfaq Hasan, M.D
Department of Pulonary Medicine,
Deccan College of Medical Sciences
Care Institute of Medical Sciences (Banjara)
Hyderabad, Andhra Pradesh
India

ISBN 978-1-4471-4314-7   ISBN 978-1-4471-4315-4   (eBook)
DOI 10.1007/978-1-4471-4315-4
Springer London Heidelberg New York Dordrecht

Library of Congress Control Number: 2013934836

Printed on acid-free paper

Springer is part of Springer Science+Business Media (www.springer.com)

To my wife

Preface to the Second Edition

One of the primary objectives of the first edition of this book was to facilitate understanding and retention of a complex subject in the least possible time—by breaking the subject matter down into small, easily comprehensible sections: these were presented in a logical sequence as flow charts, introducing concepts first, and then gradually building upon them.

The aim of the second edition is no different. However, keeping pace with the requirements of busy modern health providers, several changes have been made. Many sections have been completely rewritten and new ones added. The format is now more conventional. For better readability, the size of the print has been enlarged and made uniform throughout the book. In spite of this, the volume has been kept down to a manageable size.

My thanks are due to Liz Pope, Senior Editorial Assistant; to Grant Weston, Senior Editor, who was involved with my other books as well; to my colleague MA Aleem, for his valuable advice; and to my readers who found the time to provide valuable feedback—much of which is reflected in this second edition.

Hyderabad   Ashfaq Hasan, M.D
India

Preface to the First Edition

> *[Blood gas analysis is] the...single most helpful laboratory test in managing respiratory and metabolic disorders. [It is]... imperative to consider an ABG for virtually any symptom..., sign..., or scenario... that occurs in a clinical setting, whether it be the clinic, hospital, or ICU.[1]*

For the uninitiated, the analysis of blood gas can be a daunting task. Hapless medical students, badly constrained for time, have struggled ineffectively with Hasselbach's modification of the Henderson equation; been torn between the Copenhagen and the Boston schools of thought; and lately, been confronted with the radically different strong-ion approach of Peter Stewart.

In the modern medical practice, the multi-tasking health provider's time has become precious—and his attention span short. It is therefore important to retain focus on those aspects of clinical medicine that truly matter. In the handling of those subjects rooted in clinical physiology (and therefore predictably difficult to understand), it makes perfect sense, in my opinion, to adopt an 'algorithmic' approach. A picture can say a thousand words; a well-constructed algorithm can save at least a hundred—not to say, much precious time—and make for clarity of thinking. I have personally found this method relatively painless—and easy to assimilate. The book is set out in the form of flow charts in logical sequence, introducing and gradually building upon the underlying concepts.

The goal of this book is to enable medical students, residents, nurses and respiratory care practitioners to quickly grasp the principles underlying respiratory and acid-base physiology, and to apply the concepts effectively in clinical decision making. Each of these sections, barring a few exceptions, has been designed to fit into a single powerpoint slide: this should facilitate teaching.

---

[1] Canham EM, Beuther DA. Interpreting Arterial Blood Gases, PCCU on line, Chest.

Over the years, many excellent books and articles have appeared on the subject. I have found the manuals by Lawrence Martin[2] and Kerry Brandis[3] thoroughly enjoyable as also the online tutorials of Alan Grogono[4] and Bhavani Shankar Kodali[5]: I have tried to incorporate into my own book, some of their energy and content.

No matter how small, a project such as this can never be accomplished without the support of well wishers and friends. I would like to acknowledge the unwavering support of my colleagues Dr. TLN Swamy and Dr. Syed Mahmood Ahmed; my assistants A. Shoba and P. Sudheer; and above all, my family who had to endure the painstaking writing of yet another manuscript.

Hyderabad   Ashfaq Hasan, M.D
India

---

[2] Martin L. All you really need to know to interpret blood gases. Philadelphia: Lippincott Williams and Wilkins; 1999.

[3] Brandis K. Acid-base pHysiology; www.anaesthesiaMCQ.com

[4] Grogono AW. www.acid-base.com

[5] Kodali BS. 2007. Welcome to Capnography.com

Contents

Chapter 1
Gas Exchange

Contents

A. Hasan, *Handbook of Blood Gas/Acid-Base Interpretation*,
DOI 10.1007/978-1-4471-4315-4_1, © Springer-Verlag London 2013

1.1   The Respiratory Centre

The respiratory centre is a complex and ill-understood structure organized into 'sub-centres' that are composed of several nuclei dispersed within the medulla oblongata and pons.

The Medullary Respiratory Centres

Dorsal Respiratory Group (DRG)

The DRG consists of two groups of neurons, bilaterally, near the tractus solitarius. Axons from the DRG descend in the contralateral spinal cord and innervate the diaphragm and the inspiratory intercostal muscles. *The DRG is composed of inspiratory neurons,* the firing of which initiates inspiration.

Ventral Respiratory Group (VRG)

These are two groups of neurons bilaterally, ventromedial to the DRG, close to the nucleus ambiguus & nucleus retroambiguus. Axons from the VRG descend in the contralateral spinal cord and innervate the inspiratory and expiratory intercostals, the abdominals, the accessory muscles of respiration, and the muscles that surround the upper airway that are involved in the maintenance of airway patency. *The VRG is composed of both inspiratory and expiratory neurons.* Expiratory neurons are generally quiescent, only becoming active when the respiratory drive increases.

The Pontine Respiratory Centres

Pneumotaxis Centre

Pneumotaxis is the ability to change the rate of respiration. The function of the pneumotaxic centre is possibly to maintain a balance between inspiration and expiration.

Apneustic Centre

Stimulation of the apneustic centre results in apneusis (cessation of breathing). It can alternatively cause the prolongation of inspiration and shortening of expiration.

1.2   Rhythmicity of the Respiratory Centre

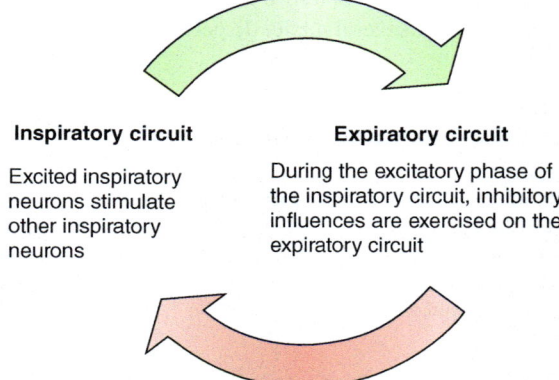

Inspiratory circuit

Excited inspiratory neurons stimulate other inspiratory neurons

Expiratory circuit

During the excitatory phase of the inspiratory circuit, inhibitory influences are exercised on the expiratory circuit

This reverberation within the inspiratory circuit dies out with fatigue of the inspiratory neurons (this takes about 2 seconds to occur), after which expiration commences. This is the reason for the rhythmicity of the respiratory centre.

Neural and chemical receptors provide vital feedback which enables the respiratory centre to regulate its output.

1.3   The Thoracic Neural Receptors

Pulmonary stretch receptors (slowly adapting)	Pulmonary stretch receptors lie within the smooth muscle of trachea & large airways and respond mainly to distension i.e., change in lung volume. Their output stops inspiration, thus limiting tidal volume (Hering-Breur reflex).
Chest wall receptors (slowly adapting)	Chest wall receptors also respond mainly to change in lung volume, and modulate respiration during exercise. They include: • Muscle spindles • Tendon organs • Receptors in costovertebral joints
Pulmonary nosiceptive receptors (rapidly adapting)	*Pulmonary irritant receptors* lie within the epithelium of the nasal mucosa, tracheobronchial tree and possibly the alveoli. They are stimulated by rapid inflation or chemical or mechanical stimulation. Stimulation of these receptors in different parts of the airway can produce different effects (in the larger airways, cough. In the small airways, tachypnea). These receptors respond distension as well as to irritant stimuli from chemical and noxious agents. *Unmyelinated C-fibers* comprise the bulk of airway nocireceptors. They also respond to irritative stimuli. Different types of C-fibres may exist, subserving different airway responses. *Juxtacapillary ('J') receptors* lie in the interstitium rather than in capillary walls. J-receptors are stimulated by vascular congestion or interstitial pulmonary edema, and result in hyperpnea.

Kubin L, Alheid GF, Zuperku EJ, McCrimmon DR. Central pathways of pulmonary and lower airway vagal afferents. J Appl Physiol. 2006;101:618.

Mazzone SB, Canning BJ. Central nervous system control of the airways: pharmacological implications. Curr Opin Pharmacol. 2002;2:220.

Undem BJ, Chuaychoo B, Lee MG, et al. Subtypes of vagal afferent C-fibres in guinea-pig lungs. J Physiol. 2004;556:905.

1.4   Chemoreceptors

Central Chemoreceptors	
Central chemoreceptors are pH$^-$ sensitive receptors located 200–500 µm below the surface of the ventrolateral medulla. They are also present in the midbrain.	*Respiratory disturbances* result in changes in $PaCO_2$. The highly lipid-soluble CO_2 diffuses rapidly across the blood-brain barrier into the CSF. As a result, *central chemoreceptors respond rapidly to respiratory disturbances.* Metabolic disturbances result in changes in serum [H$^+$] and [HCO$_3^-$]. [H$^+$] and [HCO$_3^-$] are relatively slow to equilibrate across the blood-brain barrier. As a result, *central chemoreceptors are relatively slow to respond to metabolic disturbances.*

Peripheral Chemoreceptors	
Peripheral chemoreceptors are O_2–sensitive receptors located within the carotid and aortic bodies.	See Sect. 1.6 for a more detailed discussion of peripheral chemoreceptors

Coleridge HM, Coleridge JCG. Reflexes evoked from tracheobronchial tree and lungs. In: Fishman AP, editor. Handbook of physiology. The respiratory system. Bethesda: American Physiological Society; 1986.

Lambertsen CJ. Chemical control of respiration at rest. 14th ed. St. Louis: Mosby Company; 1980.

1.5   The Central Chemoreceptors and the Alpha-Stat Hypothesis

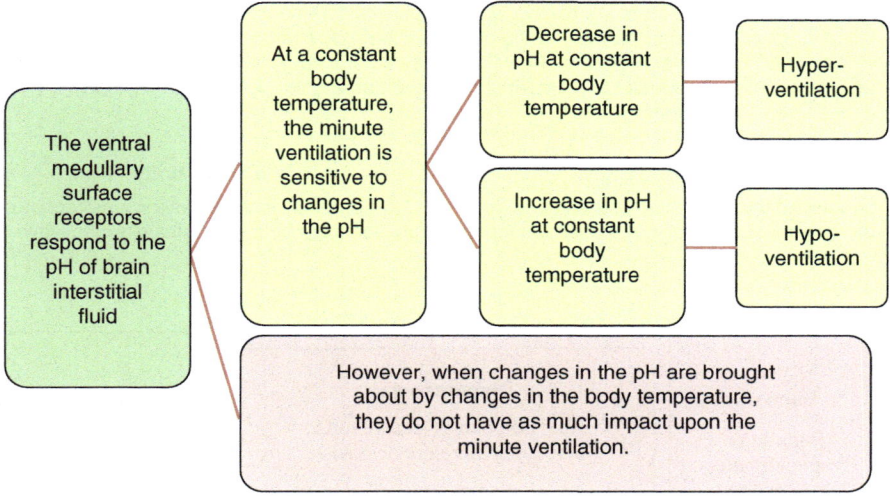

Histidine carries an imidazole moiety on its side-chain. The alpha-value of imidazole is 0.55, which means that imidazole is just over 50 % ionized; this value does not substantially change with variations of temperature. Since the ventilatory drive parallels the levels of alpha-imidazole in the local milieu and not the pH, intracellular enzymatic function remains stable in spite of temperature-related variations in pH.

The relevance of the *imidazole alpha-stat hypothesis* to the interpretation of arterial blood gases lies in that temperature-correction is not required. In contrast, the *pH-stat* based approach requires blood gas values to be first corrected to the patient's temperature, and then read off against the reference range (note that the reference range is based around a temperature of 37 °C).

This conflict has implications for patients undergoing cardiac anaesthesia: should the blood gas results of the hypothermic patient be interpreted without correction for temperature (the alpha-stat hypothesis), or should they first be corrected to the values that would prevail at a patient-temperature of 37 °C (the pH-stat hypothesis)?

Kazemi H, Johnson DC. Regulation of cerebrospinal fluid acid-base balance. Physiol Rev. 1986; 66:953.

Reeves RB. An imidazole alphastat hypothesis for vertebrate acid-base regulation: tissue carbon dioxide content and body temperature in bullfrogs. Respir Physiol. 1972;14:219–236.

1.6   Peripheral Chemoreceptors

Peripheral chemoreceptors

Peripheral chemoreceptors are composed of glomus cells, which are provided with a richer blood supply (2 litres per min, per 100 g of tissue) than any other part of the body, weight for weight. This amounts to more than forty times the cerebral blood flow. The high blood flow ensures an almost constant O_2 content of the blood passing through the glomus body, negating the effect of any anemia etc.

The carotid body

Located at the bifurcation of the carotid artery, the carotid body is the major chemoreceptor inadults.

The aortic body

Plays an important part as a chemoreceptor of infants but becomes relatively inactive in adults.

Hypoxia

Peripheral receptors are the primary sites for the 'monitoring' of PaO_2; hypoxia is their most potent stimulus

Hypercapnia

Their output can also increase with hypercapnia or acidosis.

Hypoxia and hypercapnia

A combination of these factors is a greater stimulus for their discharge than any one factor alone.

Peripheral chemo-receptors

Burton MD, Kazemi H. Neurotransmitters in central respiratory control. Respir Physiol. 2000;122:111.

Lambertsen CJ. Chemical control of respiration at rest. 14th ed. St. Louis: Mosby Company; 1980.

1.7   Chemoreceptors in Hypoxia

Peripheral chemoreceptors Hypoxia

Glomus cells synthesize and release dopamine

Dopamine stimulates post-synaptic afferent nerves within the glomus body

Carotid body	**Aortic body**
Efferents to the respiratory centre are carried through the glossopharyngeal nerve.	Efferents to the respiratory centre are carried through the vagus nerve.

Increase in minute ventilation

The mechanism underlying the direct stimulatory effect of hypoxia on *central chemoreceptors* is less well understood.

S-nitrosothiols are complexes of nitric oxide linked by a sulfhydryl group to cysteine. They are normally bound to oxygenated haemoglobin but released with deoxygenation and metabolized to S-nitroso-cysteinyl glycine by gamma-glutamyl transpeptidase. It is possible that hypoxia by causing a release of these mediators from haemoglobin, triggers a cascade of reactions that culminate in trans-nitrosylation of a cysteine residue within the nucleus tractus solitarius of the brainstem.

Coleridge HM, Coleridge JCG. Reflexes evoked from tracheobronchial tree and lungs. In: Fishman AP, editor. Handbook of physiology. The respiratory system. Bethesda: American Physiological Society; 1986.

Lipton SA. Physiology. Nitric oxide and respiration. Nature. 2001;413:118.

Lipton AJ, Johnson MA, Macdonald T, et al. S-nitrosothiols signal the ventilatory response to hypoxia. Nature. 2001;413:171.

1.8   Response of the Respiratory Centre to Hypoxemia

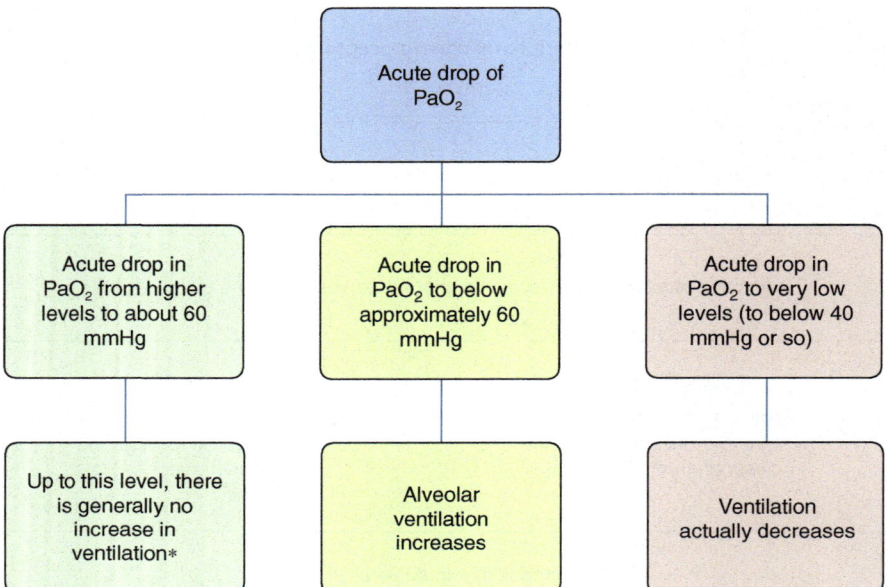

*In contrast even a small rise in CO_2 above physiological levels results in an almost immediate increase in alveolar ventilation

Igarashi T, Nishimura M, Kobayashi S, et al. Dependency on the rate of change in PaO_2 of the ventilatory response to progressive hypoxia. Am J Respir Crit Care Med. 1995;151:1815–20.

1.9   Respiration

Respiration involves the sum of those complex processes that enable gas exchange between an organism and its environment.

Ventilation	The movement of air in and out of the respiratory system (approx. 500 ml/min).	Negative intrapleural pressure created by the contraction of the respiratory muscles draws air into the respiratory zone of the lung.
Diffusion	The movement of gases (O_2 and CO_2) along pressure gradients across the alveolo-capillary membrane.	The respiratory zone of the lung comprises respiratory bronchioles, alveolar ducts and some 600 million alveoli; these are separated from the pulmonary capillaries by a 0.3μ thick alveolocapillary membrane.
Blood flow (perfusion)	The flow of blood through pulmonary capillaries (approx. 450 mL/min).	Mixed venous blood from the right ventricle flows through the pulmonary arteries to the pulmonary capillaries; oxygen enriched blood is returned to the left atrium through pulmonary veins.
Control of ventilation	Ventilation increases or decreases in response to the changing homeostatic demands of the body.	The respiratory center is an ill understood structure that lies in the brainstem. It comprises a dorsal and a ventral group of neurons, a pneumotaxic and an apneustic centre. It has been discussed in the preceding sections (see Sect. 1.1, 1.2, 1.3, 1.4, 1.5, 1.6, 1.7 and 1.8).

1.10   Partial Pressure of a Mixture of Gases

1.10.1   Atmospheric Pressure

Atmospheric pressure is essentially the weight of the atmospheric blanket of air that is pulled towards the earth by gravity. It is the sum of the pressure of all the gases present in the atmospheric air. Standard pressure is atmospheric pressure measured at sea level (1 atm).

$$1\,atm = 760\,mmHg = 14.7\,psi = 1,030\,cmH_2O$$

According to Dalton's law, the partial pressure of a gas (in a container holding a mixture of gases) is the pressure that the gas would exert if *it alone* occupied the entire volume of the given container. Within a mixture of gases, the pressure exerted by each gas is independent of the pressure exerted by all others. A given gas within a mixture behaves as though it alone were present to the exclusion of all other gases.

1.10.2   Gas Pressure

The pressure exerted by the molecules of a gas (which, above absolute zero temperature, are in a state of perpetual motion) is called the gas pressure. Gas pressure can be expressed in mmHg (millimetres of mercury), cmH_2O (centimetres of water), or psi (pounds per square inch).

$$1\,mmHg = 1,334\,dynes/cm^2 = 133.4\,Pascals$$

Partial pressure
The pressure exerted by each gas is termed its partial pressure

The pressure exerted by a mixture of gases is the sum of the individual partial pressures of the gases.

1.11   Partial Pressure of a Gas

The pressure exerted by a gas is a function of its concentration and the velocity with which its molecules move.

Partial pressure of a gas

The individual moleules of a gas by reason of the kinetic energy they possess continually vibrate, exerting a pressure on the walls of the receptacle they are contained in.
This pressure increases with:

Temperature of the gas

The higher the temperature the greater the velocity with which the molecules of the gas move; at a higher temperature, the molecules of the gas collide more often with the walls of the container.

Concentration of the gas

The greater the number of gas molecules per unit volume, the greater the number of collisions with the walls of the container; this increases the partial pressure of the gas within the container.

1.12   The Fractional Concentration of a Gas (F_{gas})

When the temperature of a gas mixture is held constant, the partial pressure of a gas is a reflection of the number of molecules of a gas (the concentration of the gas) in relation to all the molecules of the other gases present. This concentration is termed the fractional concentration of that gas (F_{gas}).

Fractional concentration and partial pressure

The fractional concentration multiplied by the total pressure gives the partial pressure of a gas.

Partial pressure of major gases in room air:

Partial pressure of Oxygen

The molecules of O_2 comprise 21 % of all the molecules in room air ($FO_2 = 0.21$).

At sea level, barometric pressure (PB) is 760 mmHg.

$PO_2 = FO_2 \times PB$
$PO_2 = 0.21 \times 760 = 159$ mmHg

Partial pressure of Nitrogen

The molecules of N_2 comprise 79 % of all the molecules in room air ($FN_2 = 0.79$).

At sea level PB is 760 mmHg.
$PN_2 = FN_2 \times PB$
$PN_2 = 0.79 \times 760 = 600$ mmHg

1.13   Diffusion of Gases

Gases always diffuse down their respective partial pressure gradients. The rate of the movement of a given gas is proportional to its partial pressure gradient.

The **net diffusion** of gases is determined by the pressure gradient of the gas. The vast majority of gas molecules move down the pressure gradient: from a region of higher pressure to a region of lower pressure (a few gas molecules do move against the pressure gradient, but their number is not significant).

The passage of gases between the alveolus and the blood are governed by the laws of simple diffusion.

Fick's Law	Graham's law	Diffusion constant
Fick's Law states that the quantity* of gas that can pass through a sheet of tissue is: *proportional to* the area (A), the diffusion constant (D) and the difference in partial pressure (P_1-P_2); *inversely proportional to* the thickness of the tissue slice (T). $V_{gas} = [(A/T) \times (P_1-P_2)] \times D/T$	Graham's law states that the rate of diffusion of a gas is inversely proportional to the square root of its molecular weight.	The diffusion constant (D) is related to the solubility (Sol) and the molecular weight (MW) of the gas: $D \propto Sol / \sqrt{MW}$

*Actually, the original Fick's law mentioned pressure, not quantity.

1.14   Henry's Law and the Solubility of a Gas in Liquid

Henry's Law states that the volume of a gas that will dissolve in a given volume of liquid is directly proportional to the partial pressure of the gas above it. In respect of water, the partial pressure of the O_2 dissolved in water (PwO_2) is directly proportional to the partial pressure of the O_2 in the gas phase (PgO_2).

The gas-liquid interface	• At a gas-liquid interface, the partial pressure of gas (e.g. O_2) **over** the liquid (e.g. water) determines the number of gas molecules **colliding** with the liquid.
Molecules entering liquid phase from the gas phase	• The number of molecules of the gas **entering** the liquid is directly proportional to partial pressure of O_2 (PgO_2) over the liquid.
Partial pressure of gases in gas phase and liquid phase	• At **equilibrium** the number of O_2 molecules entering the liquid phase (e.g. water) from the gas phase are equal to the number of O_2 molecules leaving the liquid phase and re-entering the gas phase.

1.15   Inhaled Air

Inhaled air contains virtually no CO_2; in contrast, CO_2 comprises as much as 4 % of exhaled air; the fractional concentration of N_2 of the inhaled and exhaled air is the same.

O$_2$ and CO_2 are exchanged between the alveoli and the blood by diffusion; concentration gradients determine the passage of these gases across the alveolo-capillary membrane.

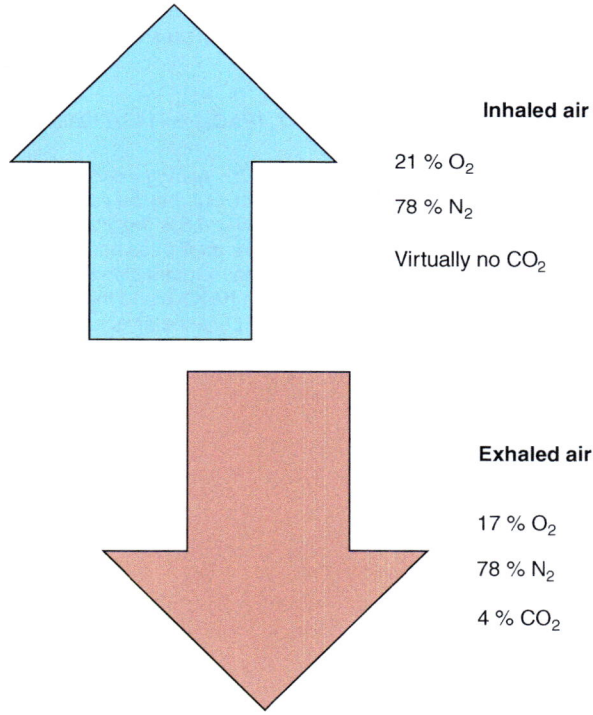

Inhaled air

21 % O_2

78 % N_2

Virtually no CO_2

Exhaled air

17 % O_2

78 % N_2

4 % CO_2

The alveolar-capillary barrier is only 0.2–0.5 μm thick. CO_2 diffuses with felicity across biological membranes. Thus, in parenchymal lung disease, even though hypoxemia may be present, CO_2 diffusion almost never presents a problem.

1.16   The O_2 Cascade

At sea level, the partial pressure of O_2 is: 760 mmHg $\times$ 0.21 = 160 mmHg

Oxygen is available for inspiration at sea level at a partial pressure of about 160 mmHg

Within the respiratory tract the partial pressure of O_2 is: 0.21 $\times$ (760–47) = 149 mmHg (or roughly 150 mmHg).

As it enters the respiratory system, O_2 is humidified by the addition of water vapour (partial pressure 47 mmHg). Humidification serves to make the inspired air more breathable; it also results in the drop of the partial pressure of oxygen to about 150 mmHg.

In the alveoli the partial pressure of O_2 (PAO_2) is: 149–(40/0.8) = 99 mmHg (or roughly about 100 mmHg)

40 is the normal value of $PaCO_2$ in mmHg. CO_2 being easily diffusible across the alveolo-capillary membrane, arterial CO_2 ($PaCO_2$) may be assumed to have the same value the same as alveolar CO_2 ($PACO_2$). 0.8 is the Respiratory Quotient. In the alveoli, oxygen diffuses into the alveolar capillaries and carbon dioxide is added to the alveolar air. The result of a complex interaction between three factors—alveolar ventilation, CO_2 production (VCO_2), and the relative consumption of O_2 (VO_2)—causes the partial pressure of O_2 in the alveolus to drop to 100 mmHg. This is the pressure of oxygen that equates with the pressure of oxygen in the pulmonary veins, and therefore, with the pressure of oxygen in the systemic arteries.

VCO_2 = 250 ml of CO_2 per minute

VO_2 = 300 ml of O_2 per minute

In the systemic arteries the partial pressure of O$_2$ (PaO$_2$) is about 95 mmHg.

A small amount of deoxygenated blood is added to the systemic arteries (because of a small physiological shunt that normally exists in the body). This is due to the unoxygenated blood that is emptied by certain systemic arteries–the bronchial and thesbesian veins–back into the pulmonary veins, and into the left side of the heart. This 'shunt fraction' which represents about 2–5 % of the cardiac output, causes the systemic arterial oxygen to fall fractionally–from 100 mmHg, to about 95 mmHg or less. Thus, in spite of normal gas exchange, the PaO$_2$ may be 5–10 mmHg lower than the PAO$_2$.

In the mitochondrion the partial pressure of O$_2$ is unknown.

Due to substantial diffusion barriers, the amount of oxygen made available to the oxygen-processing unit of the cell (the mitochondrion) is a relatively tiny amount. The mitochondrion appears to continue in its normal state of aerobic metabolism with minimal oxygen requirements. In hypoxia, a fall in the PaO$_2$ within mitochondria (to possibly less than 1 mmHg), is required to shift the energy producing pathways towards the much less efficient anaerobic metabolism.

Hasan A. Alveolar Ventilation. In: Understanding Mechanical Ventilation: a Practical Handbook. London: Springer; 2010. p. 39–46.

Hasan A. Esophageal Intubation. In: Understanding Mechanical Ventilation: a Practical Handbook. London: Springer; 2010. p. 183, 309–10.

Hasan A. Monitoring Gas Exchange. In: Understanding Mechanical Ventilation: a Practical Handbook. London: Springer; 2010. p. 149–56.

1.17 PaO$_2$

The measurement of oxygen in the blood serves as a surrogate for the measurement of oxygen in the tissues...

...there being no practical way to reliably assess the state of tissue oxygenation.

The normal level of PaO$_2$ declines with advancing age

PaO$_2$ in healthy young adults (at sea level)

Average PaO$_2$: 95 mmHg
(range 85–100 mmHg)

In a healthy 60 year-old (at sea level)

Average PaO$_2$: 83 mmHg

Predictive equation for the estimation of PaO$_2$ at (sea level) in different age groups

- PaO$_2$ = 109 − 0.43 × age in years

Sorbini CA, Grassi V, Solinas E, et al. Arterial oxygen tension in relation to age in healthy subjects. Respiration. 1968;25:3–13.

1.18   The Modified Alveolar Gas Equation

The value of PaO_2 (the partial pressure of O_2 in the arterial blood) cannot be interpreted in isolation. A PaO_2 which is low relative to the PAO_2 (the partial pressure of O_2 in alveolar air) implies a significant deficiency in the gas exchange mechanisms of the lung. The alveolar gas equation makes it possible to calculate the PAO_2. The difference between the PAO_2 (which is a calculated value) and the PaO_2 (which is measured in the laboratory) helps quantify the pulmonary pathology that is causing hypoxemia.

The partial pressure of the O_2 in the inspired air depends on the fraction of O_2 in the inspired air in relation to the barometric pressure at that altitude, and also upon the water vapour pressure (the upper airways completely saturate the inhaled air is with water).

$$PIO_2 = FIO_2 (P_b - P_w)$$

Where,
PIO_2 = Inspired PO_2
P_b = Barometric pressure
Pw = Water vapour pressure, 47 mmHg at the normal body temperature

$$PAO_2 = PIO_2 - 1.2 (PaCO_2)$$
Where,
PAO_2 = Partial pressure of O_2 in the alveolus
$PaCO_2$ = Partial pressure of CO_2 in the arterial blood. Because of the excellent diffusibility of CO_2 across biological membranes, the value of $PaCO_2$ is taken to be the same as the $PACO_2$ (the partial pressure of CO_2 in the alveolus).
0.8 is the respiratory quotient.
(Multiplying $PaCO_2$ by 1.2, of course, is the same as dividing $PaCO_2$ by 0.8).
Substituting the value of PIO_2 into the above equation,
$$PAO_2 = [FIO_2 (P_b - P_w)] - [1.2 \times PaCO_2]$$

The above abbreviated form of the equation serves well for clinical use, in place of the alveolar air equation proper which is:

$$PAO_2 = PIO_2 - (PACO_2) \times [FIO_2 + \{(1 - FIO_2) / R\}]$$

Martin L. Abbreviating the alveolar gas equation. An argument for simplicity. Respir Care. 1986;31:40–44. 23.

1.19 The Determinants of the Alveolar Gas Equation

The alveolar-arterial diffusion gradient (A-aDO$_2$) for oxygen is the difference between the partial pressure of O$_2$ in the alveolus (**PAO$_2$**) and the partial pressure of oxygen in the arterial blood (**PaO$_2$**).

$$A - aDO_2 = PAO_2 - PaO_2$$

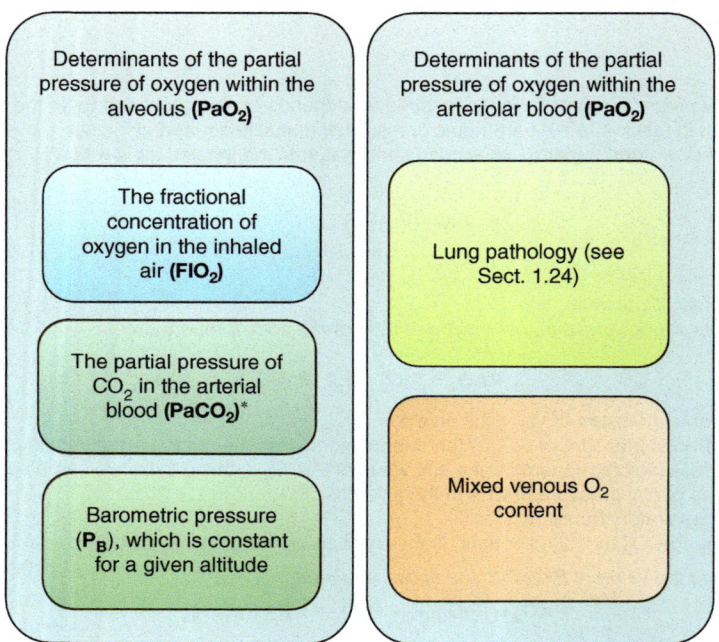

Determinants of the partial pressure of oxygen within the alveolus **(PaO$_2$)**	Determinants of the partial pressure of oxygen within the arteriolar blood **(PaO$_2$)**
The fractional concentration of oxygen in the inhaled air **(FIO$_2$)**	Lung pathology (see Sect. 1.24)
The partial pressure of CO$_2$ in the arterial blood **(PaCO$_2$)***	
Barometric pressure **(P$_B$)**, which is constant for a given altitude	Mixed venous O$_2$ content

*For reasons mentioned before, the partial pressure of CO$_2$ in the blood (PaCO$_2$) closely approximates the partial pressure of CO$_2$ in the alveolus (PACO$_2$)

1.20   The Respiratory Quotient (RQ) in the Alveolar Air Equation

RQ, for all practical purposes, equals 0.8 mathematically.

$CO_2/0.8$ can also be written as $1.2 \times CO_2$.

The respiratory quotient remains remarkably constant over a wide spectrum of clinical conditions, and therefore, in practice, the above formula usually suffices*.

The factor 1.2 may change slightly depending upon the FIO_2 administered, in order to compensate for the N_2 that is washed out with higher fractions of O_2. At FIO_2's of 100 % the factor approximates 1.0.

$FIO_2 < 0.6$	$FIO_2 > 0.6$
• Use factor 1.2**	• Use factor 1.0**
i.e.,	i.e.,
$PAO_2 = [FIO_2 (P_B-47)] - 1.2\ PaCO_2$	$PAO_2 = [FIO_2 (P_B-47)] - 1.0\ PaCO_2$

---

*Cinel D, Markwell K, Lee R, Szidon P. Variability of the respiratory gas exchange ratio during arterial puncture. Am Rev Respir Dis. 1991;143:217.

**Martin L. Abbreviating the alveolar gas equation. An argument for simplicity. Respir Care. 1986;31–40

1.21 FIO_2, PAO_2, PaO_2 and CaO_2

① The **FIO_2** (the fraction of inspired O_2) determines the **PAO_2** (the partial pressure of O_2 in the alveolus). PAO_2 is also determined by **P_B** and **$PaCO_2$** (see Sect. 2.22).

② The PAO_2 determines the **PaO_2** (partial pressure of O_2 in the pulmonary capillaries). *O_2 molecules diffuse across the alveolo-capillary membrane into the pulmonary capillaries, and equilibrate with the O_2 in the arterial blood. Thus PAO_2 determines the PaO_2 (or how much O_2 is dissolved in the plasma).*

③ **SpO_2** (O_2 saturation of the arterial blood) is determined by the **PaO_2** *The O_2 molecules in the arterial blood pass across the RBC membrane and bind to Hb. SpO_2 is the percentage of the heme sites that are bound to O_2 molecules. SpO_2 therefore is determined by the PaO_2 (or the partial pressure that O2 exerts in the blood). Generally, the higher the PaO_2, the higher the SpO_2. However this relationship is not linear* (see Sect. 2.5).

④ **CaO_2** (the O_2 content of arterial blood) is determined by the **SpO_2** and the **Hb concentration** *$CaO_2 = [1.34 \times Hb$ (in gm/dL)$^* \times SpO_2] + [PaO_2 \times 0.003$ mL O_2/mmHg]. The maximum amount of O_2 that can combine with the available Hb is termed the* **Oxygen Capacity.** *For a normal Hb of 15 gm/dL, the O_2 capacity is $= 1.34 \times 15 = 20$ mL/dL.*

(*1.34 mL of oxygen combine with each gram of Hb. 0.003 mL is the solubility of O_2 in each dL of blood per mmHg)

Hasan A. Alveolar Ventilation. In: Understanding Mechanical Ventilation: a Practical Handbook. London: Springer; 2010. p. 39–46.

Hasan A. Esophageal Intubation. In: Understanding Mechanical Ventilation: a Practical Handbook. London: Springer; 2010. p. 183, 309–10.

Hasan A. Monitoring Gas Exchange. In: Understanding Mechanical Ventilation: a Practical Handbook. London: Springer; 2010. p. 149–56.

1.22   DO$_2$, CaO$_2$, SpO$_2$, PaO$_2$ and FIO$_2$

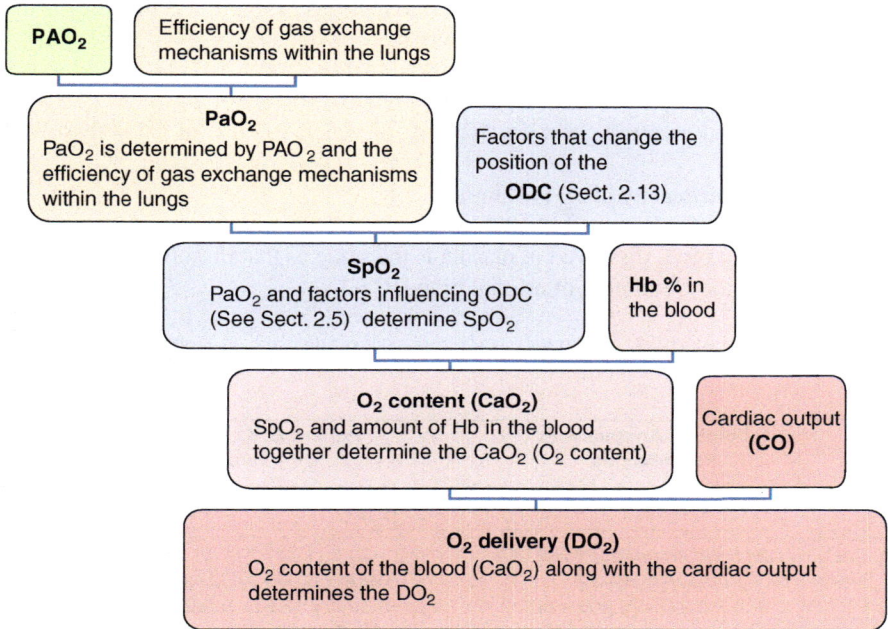

1.23 O_2 Content: An Illustrative Example

According to Henry's Law, the tension exerted by a gas in solution is the same is the tension of the gas that is in equilibrium over it.

Partial pressure of O_2 in alveolar air $= 100$ mmHg

Partial pressure of O_2 in alveolar capillary blood $= 100$ Hg

At this partial pressure, in every 100 mL of water, 0.3 mL of O_2 is dissolved (at NTP)

Given that the density of O_2 is 1.3 g/L,

The *weight* of O_2 dissolved in 100 mL water $= 0.0004$ g

The quantity of O_2 dissolved in plasma is the same as that dissolved in water.

Recall that the O_2 content of arterial blood, CaO_2

$$= [(1.34 \times Hb \text{ in gm / dL}) \times SpO_2] + [PaO_2 \times 0.003 \text{ mlO}_2 \text{ / mmHg / dL}]$$

Patient A: Anemia with normoxemia PaO_2: 90 mmHg, $SpO_2 = 97$ %, Hb: 8.5 g/dL	Patient B: COPD with chronic hypoxemia PaO_2: 58 mmHg, $SpO_2 = 88$ %, Hb: 16.5 g/dL
$CaO_2 = [1.34 \times Hb \text{ (in gm/dL)} \times SpO_2] +$ $[PaO_2 \times 0.003 \text{ mlO}_2/\text{mmHg/dL}]$ $= [(1.34 \times 8.5) \times 0.97] + [0.003 \times 90]$ $= 11.32 \text{ mLO}_2/\text{dL}$	$CaO_2 = [1.34 \times Hb \text{ (in gm/dL)} \times SpO_2] +$ $[PaO_2 \times 0.003 \text{ mlO}_2/\text{mmHg/dL}]$ $= [(1.34 \times 16.5) \times 0.88] + [0.003 \times 58]$ $= 19.62 \text{ mLO}_2/\text{dL}$

As it turns out, the PaO_2 (and therefore the dissolved O_2) contributes little to the CaO_2: one sixty-seventh of that carried by the Hb, given that the Hb level is normal.

The principal determinants of CaO_2 are Hb and SpO_2: the latter, of course is determined by PaO_2. Thus, though the PaO_2 does not seemingly contribute much to the CaO_2, it does impact the CaO_2 after all, by influencing the SpO_2.

1.24   Mechanisms of Hypoxemia

V/Q mismatch

Decreased ventilation relative to perfusion or vice versa. It is the most commonly encountered mechanism for hypoxemia (see Sect.1.38)

Shunt

An extreme form of V/Q mismatch. Due to lack of regional ventilation, unoxygenated blood returns to the left-heart, increasing the shunt fraction (see Sect.1.39).

Low barometric pressure

A decreased inspired fraction of O_2 would produce the same effect as a low barometric pressure

Hypoventilation

Decreased bulk flow in and out of the lungs. Hypoventilation leads to a buildup of CO_2 in the blood. Hypercapnia is its defining feature (see Sect.1.26).

Diffusion defect

Hypoxemia caused by a limitation of the diffusion of gas (oxygen) through the alveolar capillary membrane (see Sect.1.44).

1.25   Processes Dependent Upon Ventilation

Changes in alveolar ventilation (V_A, see Sect. 1.31) have a profound effect on $PaCO_2$. On the contrary, the relationship between V_A and PaO_2 is curvilinear: relatively large changes in V_A are required to bring about any appreciable change in PaO_2. V_A influences acid–base balance primarily through its effects on $PaCO_2$.

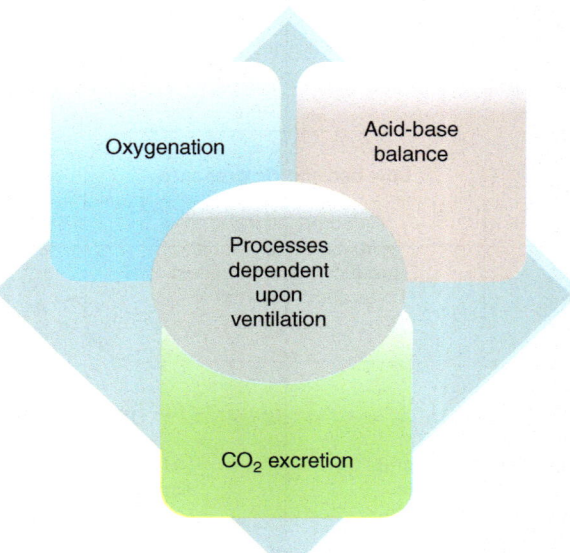

In contrast to the gradual decline in arterial PaO_2 (Sect. 1.17) that occurs with advancing age, $PaCO_2$ levels remain stable throughout life: sustained deviations in $PaCO_2$ levels from normal almost always are indicative of lung pathology.

1.26   Defining Hypercapnia (Elevated CO_2)

The value of CO_2 elevation that defines hypercapnia is not universally agreed upon. However the following are generally accepted:

$PaCO_2$ of >45 mmHg	A rise in $PaCO_2$ of >5 mmHg above baseline
In a previously normocapnic individual, a $PaCO_2$ of >45 mmHg represents the threshold for acute hypercapnia.	In a chronically hypercapnic person, a rise in $PaCO_2$ of >5 mmHg above the baseline represents acute-on-chronic hypercapnic respiratory failure.

The level of $PaCO_2$ depends on the balance between CO_2 production and CO_2 elimination.

CO_2 production	CO_2 elimination	
CO_2 production is dependent upon the rate of tissue metabolism.	CO_2 elimination is dependent upon the amount of alveolar ventilation. *CO_2 elimination is much more important at determining $PaCO_2$ than is CO_2 production.*	
CO_2 *production* almost never influences $PaCO_2$ when ventilatory mechanisms are intact. Hyperventilation or hypoventilation occurs in response to increased or decreased CO_2 respectively, tending to normalize the CO_2 levels.	**$PaCO_2$ rises when CO_2 *elimination* is low relative to CO_2 production.** A rise in $PaCO_2$ almost always implies inadequate removal of CO_2 from the circulation by the lungs, i.e., hypoventilation.	**$PaCO_2$ falls when CO_2 elimination is high relative to CO_2 production.** A fall in $PaCO_2$ almost always implies excessive washout of CO_2 from the circulation by the lungs i.e., hyperventilation.

1.27   Factors That Determine PaCO$_2$ Levels

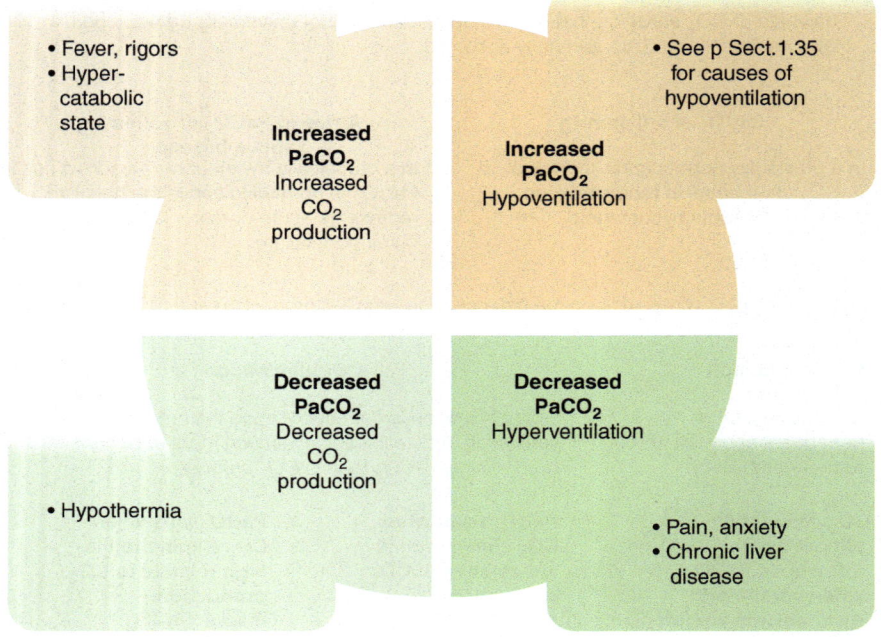

Hyperventilation (increased alveolar ventilation) results in a washout of PaCO$_2$. Hypoventilation (decreased alveolar ventilation) results in a build-up of PaCO$_2$.

1.28   Relationship Between CO$_2$ Production and Elimination

The relationship between CO$_2$ production and elimination can be summarized by the respiratory equation:

$$PaCO_2 \; \alpha \; (VCO_2 \,/\, VA)$$

Where,
VCO$_2$ = CO$_2$ production
VA = alveolar ventilation
This relationship holds true provided there is no CO$_2$ in the inhaled gas.

According to the respiratory equation, CO$_2$ will be expected to rise if:

CO$_2$ production (VCO$_2$) is increased in the face of unchanged alveolar ventilation (VA)*

Hyperthermia (for each degree Centigrade that the body temperature rises, there is approximately a 14 % increase in CO$_2$ production)

Exercise

Rigors

Alveolar ventilation (VA) decreases in the face of unchanged VCO$_2$

This may occur if:

Physiological dead space (VD/VT) increases

There is a decrease in minute ventilation

*Unchanged alveolar ventilation, as in the setting of a paralysed patient on controlled mechanical ventilation

1.29 Exercise, CO_2 Production and $PaCO_2$

During exercise there is an approximately linear increase in the respiratory rate, and a hyperbolic increase in tidal volume, and together these may produce a substantial increase in minute ventilation. In spite of this, both $PaCO_2$ and PaO_2 are maintained within narrow limits.

Increased CO_2 production:

If CO_2 production is increased *in the absence of lactic acidosis* (as in *exercise below* the anerobic threshold):

If CO_2 production is increased *with concurrent lactic acidosis* (as in exercise *above* the anerobic threshold):

CO_2 elimination increases

CO_2 elimination increases

Being physiological, the elimination of CO_2 is matched to its production.

$PaCO_2$ *is unchanged.*

However, because of the associated lactic acidosis (see Sect. 9.29),

$PaCO_2$ *falls.*

Casaburi R, Daly J, Hansen JE, et al. Abrupt changes in mixed venous blood gas composition after the onset of exercise. J Appl Physiol. 1989;67:1106.

Hansen JE, Sue DY, Wasserman K. Predicted values for clinical exercise testing. Am Rev Respir Dis. 1984;129(Suppl):S49.

Wasserman K, Whipp BJ. Exercise physiology in health and disease. Am Rev Respir Dis. 1975;112:219.

1.30   Dead Space

Anatomical dead space

The space within the conducting airways (mouth and nose down to and including the terminal bronchi). Conducting airways play no part in gas exchange. The volume of air in the adult conducting airways is approximately 150 ml.

Physiological dead space

The volume of gas within the respiratory system that is not participating in gas exchange. It consists of the sum of the **anatomical dead space** and the **alveolar dead space.**

Alveolar dead space

The space within patent but unperfused alveoli. The air within these alveoli takes no part in gas exchange. In health, the alveolar dead space is negligible, but may expand markedly in disease.

1.31   Minute Ventilation and Alveolar Ventilation

Minute ventilation (VE)	Alveolar ventilation (VA)
The total amount of air moved in and out of the lungs each minute.	The amount of air moved in and out of the lungs each minute, *that is participating in gas exchange.*
VE = Vt × f VE = Minute volume Vt = Tidal volume f = Respiratory frequency	VA = **(Vt–DS)** × f VA = VE – VD VE = Minute volume VD = Dead space volume

The difference between minute ventilation and alveolar ventilation is dead space ventilation. In the absence of physiological dead space, these terms would be synonymous.

1.32   The Determinants of the PaCO$_2$

The determinants of PaCO$_2$ can be predicted from the following equation:

$$VA = VE - VD$$

VA = alveolar ventilation
VE = minute ventilation i.e., respiratory frequency × tidal volume
VD = dead-space ventilation i.e., resp frequency × physiological dead space
   Looking at the equation above it can be appreciated that decreased VA can only be possible if *VE is low* or *VD is high.*

Decreased VE

All the conditions causing a decrease in bulk flow into the lungs (see Sect. 1.35) are capable of producing hypoventilation.

Increased VD

In clinical practice, it is an increase in *alveolar* dead space that results in the expansion of the physiological dead space.

According to the PaCO$_2$ equation,
PaCO$_2$ α VCO$_2$/VA

PaCO$_2$ = Partial pressure of CO$_2$ in the arterial blood

VCO$_2$ = CO$_2$ production in mL/min

VA   = Alveolar ventilation in L/min

PaCO$_2$ is therefore the CO$_2$ production relative to the alveolar ventilation. Since CO$_2$ production is rarely a clinically important factor, the adequacy of alveolar ventilation is the most important determinant of PaCO$_2$.

Increase in PaCO$_2$

Occurs when alveolar ventilation is low relative to CO$_2$ production.

Decrease in PaCO$_2$

Occurs when alveolar ventilation is high relative to CO$_2$ production.

Alveolar ventilation is the most important determinant of PaCO$_2$.

1.33   Alveolar Ventilation in Health and Disease

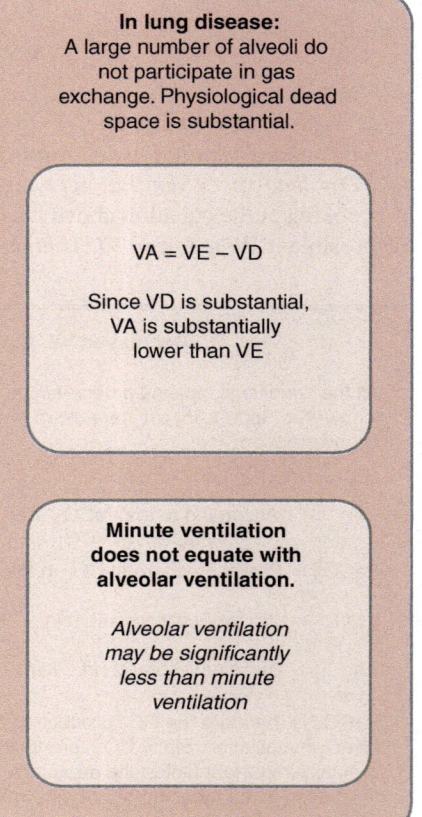

In health:
Nearly all alveoli participate in gas exchange. Physiological dead space is insignificant.

VA = VE − VD

Since VD is insignificant, VE practically equals VA

Minute ventilation roughly approximates the alveolar ventilation

In lung disease:
A large number of alveoli do not participate in gas exchange. Physiological dead space is substantial.

VA = VE − VD

Since VD is substantial, VA is substantially lower than VE

Minute ventilation does not equate with alveolar ventilation.

Alveolar ventilation may be significantly less than minute ventilation

Hasan A. Alveolar Ventilation. In: Understanding Mechanical Ventilation: a Practical Handbook. London: Springer; 2010. p. 39–46.

Hasan A. Esophageal Intubation. In: Understanding Mechanical Ventilation: a Practical Handbook. London: Springer; 2010. p. 183, 309–10.

Hasan A. Monitoring Gas Exchange. In: Understanding Mechanical Ventilation: a Practical Handbook. London: Springer; 2010. p. 149–56.

1.34   Hypoventilation and PaCO$_2$

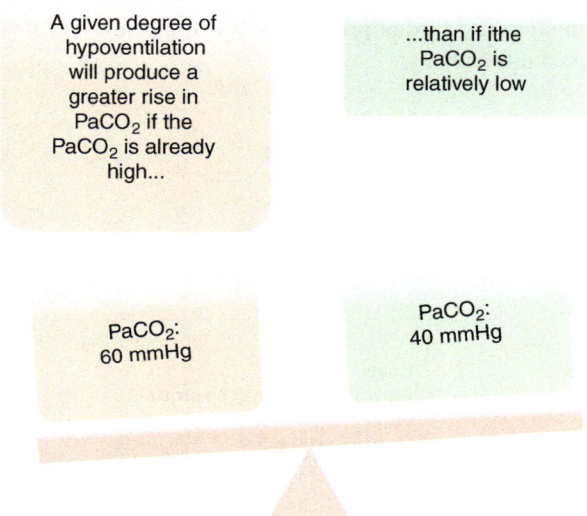

A given degree of hypoventilation will produce a greater rise in PaCO$_2$ if the PaCO$_2$ is already high...

...than if ithe PaCO$_2$ is relatively low

PaCO$_2$: 60 mmHg

PaCO$_2$: 40 mmHg

When the PaCO$_2$ is normal,

...it takes relatively large changes in alveolar ventilation to produce significant changes in PaCO$_2$

When the PaCO$_2$ is high,

... small changes in alveolar ventilation will cause proportionately great changes in PaCO$_2$

Because of the reciprocal relation between alveolar PO$_2$ and PCO$_2$, a rise in PACO$_2$ will result in a drop in PAO$_2$, and the hypoxemia will be commensurately severe with increasing levels of CO$_2$.

1.35 The Causes of Hypoventilation

Hypoventilation results from decreased bulk-flow in and out of the lungs.

Inspiration results in the bulk flow of air into the lungs, up to the level of the smallest bronchioles. The further progress of gas molecules occurs by the mechanism of facilitated diffusion.

CNS depression	Sedative agents Cerebrovascular accidents Central sleep apnea Metabolic alkalosis Myxedema Hyperoxia (Hyperoxic hypoventilation)
Spinal cord or peripheral nerve disorders	Spinal trauma Amyotrophic lateral sclerosis Polio Multiple sclerosis Guillian Barre syndrome Botulism
Neuro-muscular disorders	Aminoglycosides Paralysing agents Steroid myopathy Myasthenia gravis Muscular dystrophies Dyselectrolytemias Poor nutrition Respiratory muscle fatigue
Disorders affecting the thoracic Cage	Kyphoscoliosis Flail chest Ankylosing spondylosis
Proximal airway (extra-pulmonary airway) obstruction	Tracheal obstruction by stenosis, tumor etc. Epiglottitis Obstructive sleep apnea

Severe intrapulmonary derangements such as tight airway obstruction in COPD and asthma are also capable of producing hypoventilation by increasing physiological dead space and thereby increasing the $PaCO_2$.

1.36   Blood Gases in Hypoventilation

Hypoventilation (type 2 respiratory failure)

Hypoventilation may exist as an isolated abnormality, or there may be an additional mechanism of hypoxemia accompanying it.

'Pure' hypoventilation

Here the gas-exchange mechanism of the lungs is intact, and hypoventilation (i.e., reduction of bulk airflow) is the sole cause for the hypoxemia

Hypoventilation assaociated with an additional mechanism of hypoxemia

---

Rise in $PaCO_2$ approximately matches the fall in PaO_2.

The PaO_2 falls about 1.25 mmHg for every 1 mmHg rise in $PaCO_2$.

$A\text{-}aDO_2$ is normal.

Fall in PaO_2 is disproportionate to the rise in $PaCO_2$

$A\text{-}aDO_2$ is widened

1.37   Decreased CO_2 Production

Although increasing alveolar ventilation is the preferred method of decreasing $PaCO_2$ levels, on occasion it becomes necessary to decrease CO_2 production (such as in severe hypoxemia). By decreasing the work of breathing and metabolic rate (for instance, by sedating a patient on mechanical ventilation) a decrease in $PaCO_2$ can often be achieved. Recall that a decrease in $PaCO_2$ will reciprocally increase PO_2 (Sect. 1.36). In a borderline situation this often enables delivery of a lower FIO_2 (thereby avoiding O_2 toxicity), and allows delivery of smaller tidal volumes (thereby avoiding alveolar overdistension and volutrauma).

1.37.1   Summary: Conditions That Can Result in Hypercapnia

In summary, the conditions in which $PaCO_2$ can be increased are:

Increased proportion of CO_2 in inspired air
Rebreathing of air
Laparoscopic insufflation of air into the body

Increased production of CO_2, e.g.
Hypercatabolic states: sepsis, malignant hyperthermia, etc.

Decreased alveolar ventilation
By far the most important cause.

Increased physiological dead space
Usually occurs as a result of an increase in alveolar dead space.

Hasan A. Alveolar Ventilation. In: Understanding Mechanical Ventilation: a Practical Handbook. London: Springer; 2010. p. 39–46.

Hasan A. Esophageal Intubation. In: Understanding Mechanical Ventilation: a Practical Handbook. London: Springer; 2010. p.183, 309–10.

Hasan A. Monitoring Gas Exchange. In: Understanding Mechanical Ventilation: a Practical Handbook. London: Springer; 2010. p. 149–56.

1.38   V/Q Mismatch: A Hypothetical Model

Types of V/Q mismatch:
  Low V/Q mismatch: Ventilation low relative to perfusion
  High V/Q mismatch: Perfusion low relative to ventilation

Assume that the normal minute ventilation to both lungs: 2v.
Assume that the normal perfusion to both lungs: 2q

The Right Lung accounts for half of the total ventilation and half of the total perfusion
  Ventilation to the right lung = v
  Perfusion to the right lung = q

The Left Lung account for half of the total ventilation and half of the total perfusion.
  Ventilation to the left lung = v
  Perfusion to the left lung = q

Now assume that the ventilation of the right lung is artificially reduced to zero, and that the perfusion of the right lung is doubled

  Ventilation = 0
  Perfusion = 2q

Assume that the ventilation of the left lung is doubled, and that the perfusion of the left lung is reduced to zero.

  Ventilation = 2v
  Perfusion = 0

Therefore, the total minute ventilation to *both* lungs:
  = 2v (which is normal)
And the total perfusion to *both* lungs:
  = 2q (this is normal too)

Yet there is complete mismatching of ventilation to perfusion! None of the air ventilating the lungs comes into contact with the blood perfusing it, and life is not possible on account of hypoxemia.

Right lung:
Ventilation = 0
Perfusion = 2q
V/Q ratio = 0/2q = zero

Left lung:
Ventilation = 2v
Perfusion = zero
V/Q ratio = 2v/0 = Infinity

This is an example of an extreme **low V/Q mismatch, i.e., the right to left shunt.**

This is an example of an extreme **high V/Q mismatch, i.e. dead space ventilation.**

Forster II RE, DuBois AB, Briscoe WA, Fisher AB. The lung: physiological basis of pulmonary function tests. Chicago: Year Book Medical Publishers, Inc.; 1986.

1.39   V/Q Mismatch and Shunt

Low V/Q mismatch is the commonest mechanism of hypoxemia.

A right to left shunt is an extreme example of a low V/Q mismatch. The V/Q ratio is zero.

Etiology of right to left shunt

ARDS
Cardiogenic pulmonary edema
Lobar pneumonia
Atelectasis
Pulmonary thromboembolism (here, a shunt occurs by the reflex closure of alveoli)
Pulmonary arterio-venous malformations
Intracardiac right-to-left shunts

The administration of 100 % O_2 enables differentiation between a low V/Q mismatch and shunt

Low V/Q mismatch: Ventilation reduced relative to perfusion	**Shunt:** No ventilation, intact perfusion
Supplemental O_2 (FIO_2 1.0) eventually reaches the poorly ventilated alveoli	Supplemental O_2 (FIO_2 1.0) cannot reach the obliterated alveoli
PaO_2 rises	*PaO_2 does not rise*

1.40 Quantifying Hypoxemia

Multiplying FIO_2 into 5, gives the approximate expected PaO_2 for the given FIO_2 (provided that the gas exchange mechanisms within the lungs are normal)	• Eg, if the FIO_2 is 21 % (as in a person breathing room air) the expected $PaO_2 = 21 \times 5 = 105$ (approximately). • Similarly breathing 50 % O_2 (FIO_2 0.5) would result in an expected PaO_2 of roughly $50 \times 5 = 250$. • If the measured PaO_2 is significantly below the expected PaO_2, there is a problem with the gas exchange .
The PaO_2:FIO_2 ratio This (P:F ratio) makes it possible to compare the arterial oxygenation of patients breathing different FIO_2's.	• A normal person breathing room air would have a PaO_2 of approximately 100 mm Hg. The PaO_2/FIO_2 would be: 100/0.21 = 500. • The normal range for the PaO_2/FIO_2 ratio is 300–500. • In the appropriate setting a P:F ratio of less than 300 indicates acute lung injury (ALI) while a P:F ratio of less than 200 is diagnostic of ARDS in the appropriate setting.
The PaO_2/PAO_2 ratio A better estimate of oxygenation than the P:F ratio.	• The PaO_2 is obtained from the ABG • The PAO_2 cannot be directly measured at the bedside and needs to be calculated from the modified alveolar air equation (see Sect. 1.42) • PaO_2/PAO_2 ratio offers better accuracy over a broader range of FIO_2 than the PF ratio.

Bernard GR, Artigas A, Brigham KL, et al. The American European Consensus Conference on ARDS: definitions, mechanisms, relevant outcomes and clinical trial coordination. Am J Respir Crit Care Med. 1994;149:818–24.

Covelli HD, Nessan VJ, Tuttle WK. Oxygen derived variables in acute respiratory failure. Crit Care Med. 1983;8:646.

Peris LV, Boix JH, Salom JV, et al. Clinical use of the arterial/alveolar oxygen tension ratio. Crit Care Med. 1983;11:888.

1.41   Compensation for Regional V/Q Inequalities

Hypoperfusion an alveolus	Hypoventilation of an alveolus
High V/Q mismatch	*Regional hypoxia*
CO_2 which normally diffuses easily from the alveolar capillary blood into the alveolus cannot now as easily do so.	Hypoxic vasoconstriction
Partial pressure of CO_2 within the alveolus falls from its normal 40 mmHg.	
Hypocapnia within the alveolus causes reflex regional closure of the under-perfused alveolus.	Perfusion now becomes matched to ventilation, the V/Q mismatching decreases and hypoxemia is minimized.
Ventilation now becomes matched to perfusion. V/Q mismatching (and therefore the hypoxemia) is minimized.	

1.42   Alveolo-Arterial Diffusion of Oxygen (A-aDO$_2$)

The A-aDO$_2$ is the difference between the alveolar O$_2$ tension (PAO$_2$) and the arterial oxygen tension (PaO$_2$). A-aDO$_2$ represents the ease with which the inspired oxygen diffuses into the blood, and therefore reflects the efficiency of the lungs in oxygenating the blood. In order to estimate the A-aDO$_2$ it is necessary to calculate the PAO$_2$ (from the modified alveolar gas equation):

$$PAO_2 = FIO_2(P_b - P_w) - PaCo_2 / R$$

where,

PAO$_2$ = alveolar oxygen tension
FIO$_2$ = fraction of inspired oxygen
P$_b$ = atmospheric pressure in mmHg
P$_w$ = partial pressure of water (47 mmHg at body temperature)
PaCO$_2$ = arterial CO$_2$ tension
R = respiratory quotient

LIMITATIONS OF THE SIMPLIFIED FORMULA IN A-aDO$_2$ CALCULATION	
FIO$_2$	The estimate of the precise FIO$_2$ that the patient is breathing, is often inaccurate. Variable performance devices like nasal prongs and non-venturi masks provide unreliable estimates of FIO$_2$.
	FIO$_2$ estimates can be misleading on conventional oxygen devices if a patient has an irregular pattern of breathing.
P$_B$	The barometric pressure does not remain constant throughout the day though it is invariably assumed to be.
P$_w$	Water vapour pressure is assumed to be 47 mmHg: actually, the water vapor pressure changes slightly with body temperature.
R	The respiratory quotient is not always 0.8, especially in critically ill patients with altered body metabolism and on complex nutritive supplementation.

Kanber GJ, King FW, Eshchar YR, Sharp JT. The alveolar-arterial oxygen gradient in young and elderly men during air and oxygen breathing. Am Rev Respir Dis. 1968;97:376.

Martin L. All you really need to know to interpret blood gases. Philadelphia: Lippincott Williams and Wilkins; 1999. p. 53.

Mellemgaard, K. The alveolar-arterial oxygen difference: its size and components in normal man. Acta Physiol Scand. 1966;67:10.

1.43   A-aDO$_2$ is Difficult to Predict on Intermediate Levels of FIO$_2$

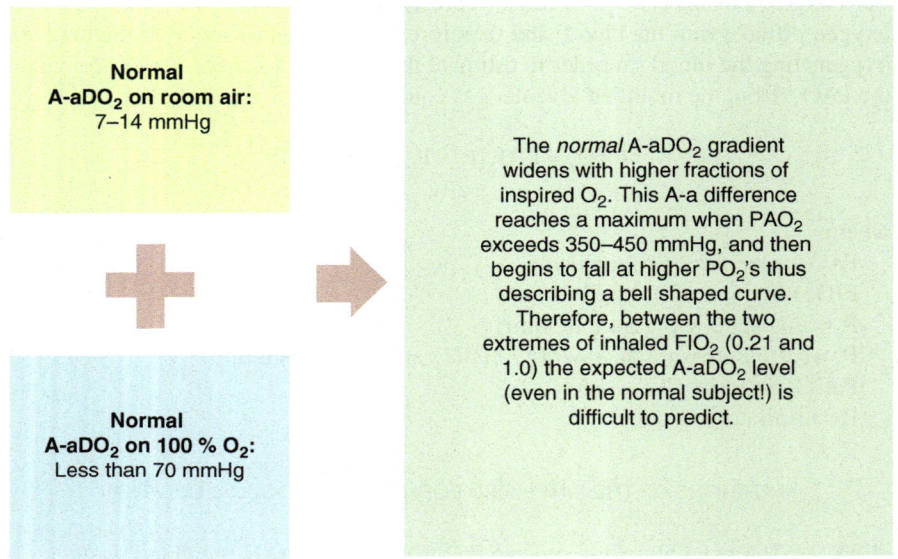

Normal A-aDO$_2$ on room air: 7–14 mmHg

Normal A-aDO$_2$ on 100 % O$_2$: Less than 70 mmHg

The *normal* A-aDO$_2$ gradient widens with higher fractions of inspired O$_2$. This A-a difference reaches a maximum when PAO$_2$ exceeds 350–450 mmHg, and then begins to fall at higher PO$_2$'s thus describing a bell shaped curve. Therefore, between the two extremes of inhaled FIO$_2$ (0.21 and 1.0) the expected A-aDO$_2$ level (even in the normal subject!) is difficult to predict.

The A-aDO$_2$ normally increases with age. The following formula predicts the A-aDO$_2$ for a given age:

$$A\text{-}aDO_2 = 2.5 + (0.25 \times Age\ in\ years)$$

Gilbert R, Keighley JF. The arterial/alveolar oxygen tension ratio. An index of gas exchange applicable to varying inspired oxygen concentrations. Am Rev Respir Dis. 1974;109:142.

Kanber GJ, King FW, Eshchar YR, Sharp JT. The alveolar-arterial oxygen gradient in young and elderly men during air and oxygen breathing. Am Rev Respir Dis. 1968;97:376.

1.44   Defects of Diffusion

In health, the PaO_2 of capillary blood equilibrates with the alveolar gas in approximately 0.25 seconds.
This is more than enough time for adequate oxygenation of the RBC, since the RBC spends 0.75 seconds in the pulmonary capillaries. It has been estimated that the circulation time would prove insufficient for the oxygenation of the RBC when heart rates exceed 240 beats/min.

Disorders causing diffusion defects* such as interstitial processes retard the diffusion of oxygen into the blood. There is now not enough time for the oxygenation of the Hb within RBCs especially during exercise when the circulation time is rapid.

Like the other causes of hypoxemia (other than shunt), a diffusion defect can be easily corrected by administration of supplemental oxygen.
A diffusion defect is a relatively unusual mechanism of hypoxemia in ICU patients

*Interstitial fibrosis is the classical cause for a diffusion defect, but even in this condition, it is a V/Q mismatch which is the primary mechanism for the hypoxemia

West JB. Pulmonary pathophysiology: the essentials. 6th ed. Philadelphia: Lippincott Williams and Wilkins; 2003. p. 22–4.

1.45   Determinants of Diffusion: DL_{CO}

The ability the lungs to transfer oxygen from inspired air to the haemoglobin across the alveolo-capillary membrane (ACM) is measured by the DL_{CO}. Carbon monoxide (CO) has an incredibly high avidity for Hb. Also, its uptake is not affected by the pulmonary blood flow. This makes the test less vulnerable to variations in the cardiac output.

Alveolo-capillary membrane: Area and thickness*	**Physiologic factors** *Height:* the taller the individual the greater the lung height, and therefore, the greater the surface area of the ACM.
	Pathological factors *ILD:* (increased thickness of the ACM) *Pneumonectomy* (decrease in absolute surface area of the ACM) *Pulmonary edema* (increased "distance for diffusion") *Emphysema* (destruction and loss of the ACM; other factors also play a role in emphysema).
Pulmonary capillary blood volume: The "reservoir" of hemoglobin that exists within the pulmonary capillaries	**Physiologic factors** *Position:* increased venous return in the supine posture results in an expansion of the pulmonary capillary bed; DL_{CO} increases in the supine position. *Exercise:* increase pulmonary blood flow during exercise increases the DL_{CO}.
	Pathologic factor *Pulmonary embolism* *Pulmonary artery hypertension* *Vasculitis* *Severe emphysema*
Technical aspects: θ, the rate at which CO combines with hemoglobin	Since CO and O_2 compete for the same sites on the Hb molecule, altering the concentration of O_2 alters the rate of combination of CO with Hb (θ). V/Q mismatching affects the DL_{CO}.

*There is now evidence that the decreases in DL_{CO} may be less dependent on a decreased surface area of the alveolo-capillary membrane and more on the reduction of the red cell mass within the pulmonary circulation than earlier thought.

Enright PL. Diffusing capacity for carbon monoxide. In: Basow DS, editor. UpToDate. Waltham: UpToDate; 2012. Last updated 11 Oct 2010. Last accessed 13 May 2012.

1.46   Timing the ABG

Healthy lungs
- There is rapid mixing of inhaled air, between the different regions of the lung.

- Blood gases drawn after 5–7 min of any change in FIO_2 are acceptable.

Presence of significant lung disease
- There is slow mixing of alveolar gas because of inhomogeneity of ventilation between diseased and healthy alveolar units.

- Blood gases should ideally be drawn after 20–25 min of any change in FIO_2 to enable equilibration with those lung areas having low V/Q ratios.

Cugell DW. How long should you wait? [editorial] Chest. 1975;67:253.

1.47 A-aDO$_2$ Helps in Differentiating Between the Different Mechanisms of Hypoxemia

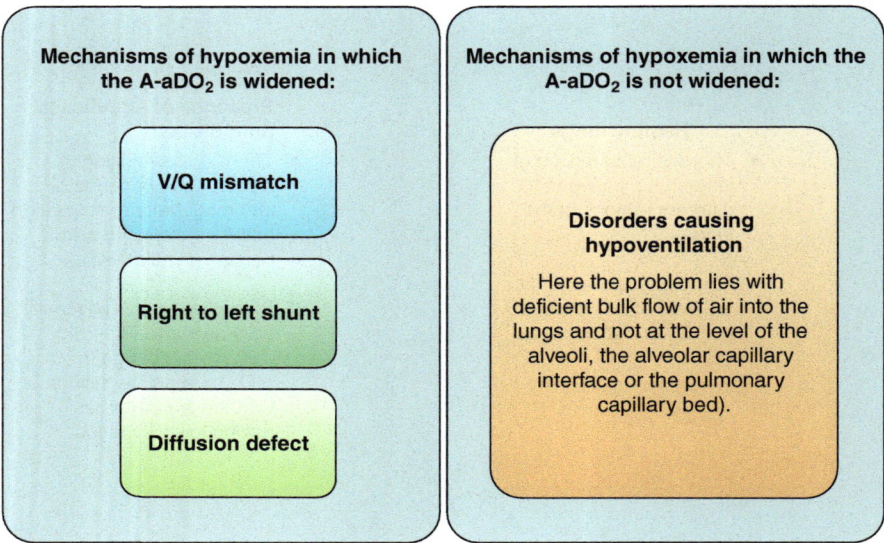

Mechanisms of hypoxemia in which the A-aDO$_2$ is widened:

- V/Q mismatch
- Right to left shunt
- Diffusion defect

Mechanisms of hypoxemia in which the A-aDO$_2$ is not widened:

Disorders causing hypoventilation

Here the problem lies with deficient bulk flow of air into the lungs and not at the level of the alveoli, the alveolar capillary interface or the pulmonary capillary bed).

Chapter 2
The Non-Invasive Monitoring of Blood Oxygen and Carbon Dioxide Levels

2

Contents

A. Hasan, *Handbook of Blood Gas/Acid-Base Interpretation*,
DOI 10.1007/978-1-4471-4315-4_2, © Springer-Verlag London 2013

2

2.1   The Structure and Function of Haemoglobin

The special ability of hemoglobin (Hb) to imbibe O_2 from the pulmonary capillaries and release it to the tissues derives from its unique quartenary structure.

Structure

Globin
The Hb molecule consists of four globin chains (two alpha chains, each of 141 amino acids; two beta chains each of 146 amino acids.

Heme
One heme group binds *each* globin chain. *Each heme group consists of:*

One ferrous ion (Fe++)	**One protoporphyrin IX ring**
In order to carry O_2, it is necessary for heme's ferrous iron to remain in the ferrous state.	This protoporphyrin ring is covalently bound to the ferrous ion.

FUNCTION: O_2 carriage is the most important function of Hb (Sect. 2.4), but Hb serves several other important functions as well:

CO_2 carriage	**Regulation of vasomotor tone**
Although only about 5 % of all the CO_2 transported in the blood is in the form of carbamino compounds (viz, bound to Hb, the latter account for 30 % of the CO_2 that evolves in the lungs from the red blood cells circulating within the pulmonary capliiaries. Another 5 % of CO_2 is carried dissolved in plasma. The bulk of the CO_2, however, is carried in the form of bicarbonate.	Nitric oxide (NO) is capable of reacting with a cysteine residue at position 93 of the ß chain of Hb. The resulting nitrosothiol, S-nitrosylated Hb is a vasodilator. The unique and recently recognized vasodilator property of Hb is dependent on its complex and ill-understood reactions with NO.

Bunn HF, Forget BG. Hemoglobin: molecular, genetic and clinical aspects. Philadelphia: WB Saunders; 1986.

McMahon TJ, Moon RE, Luschinger BP, Carraway MS, Stone AE, Stolp BW, Gow AJ, Pawloski JR, Watke P, Singel DJ, et al. Nitric oxide in the human respiratory cycle. Nat Med. 2002;8:711–7.

Perutz MF. Molecular anatomy, physiology, and pathology of hemoglobin. In: Stamatoyannopoulos G, Nienhuis AW, et al., editors. The molecular basis of blood disorders. Philadelphia: WB Saunders; 1987.

Stamler JS, Jia L, Eu JP, McMahon TJ, Demchenko IT, Bonaventura J, Gernert K, Piantadosi CA. Blood flow regulation by S-nitrosohemoglobin in the physiological oxygen gradient. Science. 1997;276:2034–7.

2.2　Co-operativity

2

Deoxygenated Hemoglobin

Deoxygenated hemoglobin exists in a tense (taut) configuration because of electrostatic bonds between its beta globin chains. The hemoglobin molecule has helical twists. In the non-helical sections the polypeptide chain folds upon itself, creating clefts within which the four heme groups lie at equidistant intervals.

The attachment of the first O_2 molecule

In its taut state, deoxygenated hemoglobin has little affinity for O_2. The attachment of the first O_2 molecule to one of the globin chains generates chemical and mechanical stresses resulting in the severing of electrostatic bonds. This allows the hemoglobin molecule to unfold slightly.

The attachment of the second O_2 molecule

As the hemoglobin molecule relaxes and unfolds it exposes the other O_2 binding sites within its clefts; this facilitates the addition of another molecule of O_2 to the hemoglobin, more rapidly than the first.

The attachment of the third and fourth O_2 molecules

The binding of the second molecule of O_2 results in further relaxation of the coils of the hemoglobin molecule, accelerating the uptake of the third and the fourth O_2 molecules.

The co-operativity among its binding sites that results in the accelerated uptake of O_2 gives the oxy-hemoglobin dissociation curve its characteristic sigmoid shape.

Bunn HF, Forget BG. Hemoglobin: molecular, genetic and clinical aspects. Philadelphia: WB Saunders; 1986.

Perutz MF. Molecular anatomy, physiology, and pathology of hemoglobin. In: Stamatoyannopoulos G, Nienhuis AW, et al. editors. The molecular basis of blood disorders. Philadelphia: WB Saunders; 1987.

2.3   The Bohr Effect and the Haldane Effect

2

Tissue capillaries
The CO_2 exiting the tissues enters the red blood corpuscles

CO_2 binding to globin and its transport as carbamino-Hb

CO_2 binds to an amino terminus of globin chain forming carbamino-Hb; 10 % of all CO_2 is transported in this form.

CO_2 transport as bicarbonate

$$CO_2 + H_2O \rightleftharpoons H_2CO_3 \rightleftharpoons HCO_3^- + H^+$$

80 % of CO_2 is transported as bicarbonate. At the peripheral tissues oxygen is already being unloaded from hemoglobin. The deoxy-Hb (which is a superior to oxy-Hb as a proton acceptor) binds the H^+ generated in the above reaction to its globin chains

Hemoglobin becomes stabilized in T-state: the CO_2-Bohr effect

Hemoglobin becomes stabilized in T-(state): the acid-Bohr effect

The Bohr effect
The Bohr effect is the CO_2– produced rightward shift of the ODC. This facilitates O_2 unloading to the tissues. The effect of CO_2 on the ODC is mostly on account of the decrease in pH that CO_2

The Haldane effect
O_2 unloading favors CO_2 uptake by hemoglobin by the Haldane effect. The CO_2 can then be transported to the lungs.

Bohr C, Hasselbalch K, Krogh A. Ueber einen in biologischer Beziehung wichtigen Einfluss. den die Kohlen- saeuerespannung des Blutes auf dessen Sauerstoffbinding ubt. Skand Arch Physiol. 1904;16:402.

Klocke RA. Mechanism and kinetics of the Haldane effect in human erythrocytes. J Appl Physiol. 1973;35:673–81.

2.4   Oxygenated and Non-oxygenated Hemoglobin

Oxygenated Hb (syn: OxyHb)	Each Hb molecule has four heme sites to each of which an O_2 molecule can bind. *The percentage of O_2 binding heme sites that bind to O_2 is the O_2 saturation (SpO_2) of the blood.* In other words SpO_2 is the number of heme sites occupied by O_2 of every 100 heme sites.	The SpO_2 (as read out on the pulse oximeter (represents) the Oxy-Hb
Non oxygenated Hb	The percentage of heme sites that are not bound to O_2 molecules. Non-oxygenated Hb includes:	**Dexoxy-Hb (syn:reduced) Hb** The percentage of heme groups that are not bound to O_2. Reduced Hb % = 100 % $-$ [SPO$_2$ + MetHb + COHb] %*
		Carboxy-Hb The percentage of heme groups in the form of Carboxy-Hb
		Met-Hb The percentage of heme groups in the form of Met-Hb

*See Co-oximetry (Sect. 2.10)

2.5 PaO$_2$ and the Oxy-hemoglobin Dissociation Curve

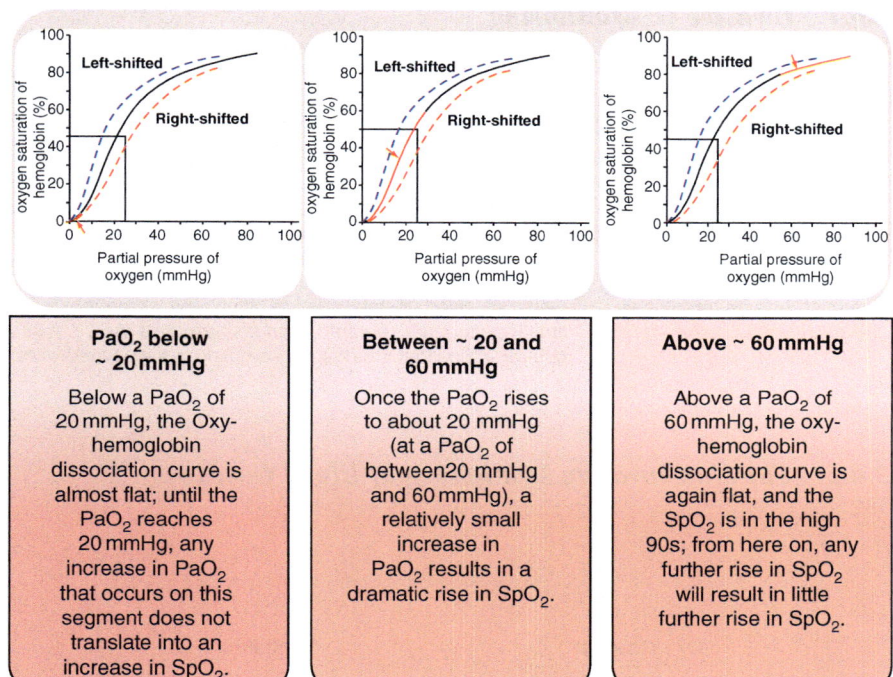

PaO$_2$ below ~ 20 mmHg	Between ~ 20 and 60 mmHg	Above ~ 60 mmHg
Below a PaO$_2$ of 20 mmHg, the Oxy-hemoglobin dissociation curve is almost flat; until the PaO$_2$ reaches 20 mmHg, any increase in PaO$_2$ that occurs on this segment does not translate into an increase in SpO$_2$.	Once the PaO$_2$ rises to about 20 mmHg (at a PaO$_2$ of between20 mmHg and 60 mmHg), a relatively small increase in PaO$_2$ results in a dramatic rise in SpO$_2$.	Above a PaO$_2$ of 60 mmHg, the oxy-hemoglobin dissociation curve is again flat, and the SpO$_2$ is in the high 90s; from here on, any further rise in SpO$_2$ will result in little further rise in SpO$_2$.

The following co-ordination points should be expected for an ODC that lies in its normal position:

PaO$_2$ 40 mmHg[*]	PaO$_2$ of 70 mmHg	PaO$_2$ of 100 mmHg
Corresponds to SpO$_2$ of 75 %	Corresponds to SpO$_2$ of 92 %	Corresponds to SpO$_2$ of 97 %

(*As in mixed venous blood)

Canham EM, Beuther DA. Interpreting arterial blood gases. Chest. 2007. PCCSU Article. 2 Jan 2007.

2

2.6   Monitoring of Blood Gases

2.6.1   *Invasive O₂ Monitoring*

Although direct measurement of arterial O_2 tension by arterial blood gas (ABG) sampling is a very accurate way of assessing oxygenation, it has its disadvantages.

Intermittent ABG sampling	Continous ABG sampling
Inconvenient Painful Blending Infection Arterial thrombosis Rarely, gangrene of extremity	Obviates the need for frequent arterial Punctures Generally used unstable clinical Situations where real time monitoring is required. *Can also produce the complications* that intermittent sampling is associated with.

2.6.2   *The Non-invasive Monitoring of Blood Gases*

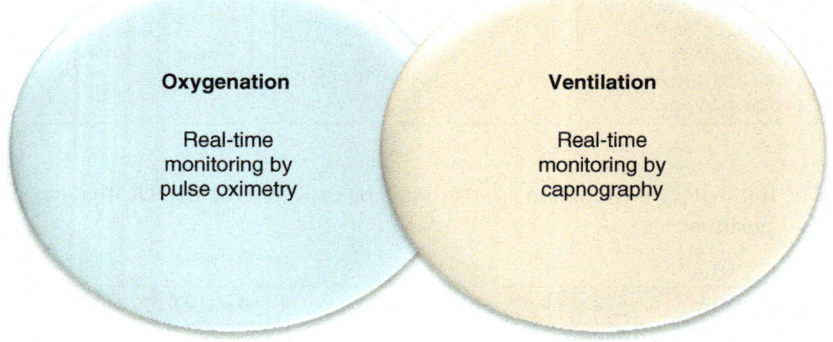

Oxygenation

Real-time monitoring by pulse oximetry

Ventilation

Real-time monitoring by capnography

Though it offers a convenient way of monitoring oxygenation in real time, pulse oximetry has its own disadvantages (Sect. 2.21).

Bongard F, Sue D. Pulse oximetry and capnography in intensive and transitional care units. West J Med. 1992;156:57.

Pierson DJ. Pulse oximetry versus arterial blood gas specimens in long-term oxygen therapy. Lung. 1990;168 Suppl:782.

2.7 Principles of Pulse Oximetry

2

Cyanosis is the *clinical* hallmark of hemoglobin desaturation.

Cyanosis is not always easy to assess at the bedside	• In an anemic patient cyanosis may be notoriously difficult to recognize.
Cyanosis requires deoxygenated Hb to fall to 5 g/dl.	• In severe anemia, not enough Hb may be available for deoxy-Hb to reach this level.

Severe hypoxia can therefore manifest without apparent cyanosis.

Pulse oximetry, which does not suffer from these limitations, has been described as "…the greatest advance in patient monitoring since electrography" and is today regarded as the "fifth vital sign".

Older oximeters calculated the SpO_2 from the values of PaO_2 and pH, deriving values through nomograms and the Severinghaus slide rule.

Modern pulse oximetry is based upon two fundamental principles:

The principle of spectro-photometry	• Used for measuring the percentages of oxyhemoglobin and deoxyhemoglobin in the blood
The principle of optical plethysmography	• Used to display the amplitude of pulse and the heart rate

---

Comroe JH Jr, Botelho S. The unreliability of cyanosis in the recognition of arterial hpoxemia. Am J Med Sci. 1947;214:1.

Hanning CD, Alexander-Williams JM. Fortnightly review: pulse oximetry: a practical review. BMJ. 1995;311:367–70.

Neff TA. Routine oximetry: a fifth vital sign? Chest. 1988;94:227.

2.8   Spectrophotometry

The principle of spectrophotometry is based upon on the *Beer-Lambert law* which states that "...*the concentration of light-absorbing species within a sample is a logarithmic function of the amount of light absorbed by that sample.*"

In respect of blood, the light-absorbing species are oxy-hemoglobin and deoxy-hemoglobin.

> Two photodiodes emit light phasically at several hundred times per second, one at 660 nm (in the red band of the spectrum) and the other at 940 nm (in the infra-red band of the spectrum).

Oxyhemoglobin	Deoxyhemoglobin
Light emitted at 660 nm is better absorbed by saturated (oxygenated) haemoglobin. *Oxygenated (red blood) absorbs light maximally in the infrared band.*	Light emitted at 940 nm is better absorbed by reduced (deoxygenated) haemoglobin. *Deoxygenated (blue blood) absorbs light maximally in the red band.*

By making the diodes blink rapidly, it is possible to make about 600 measurements each second. The relative amount of light transmitted through the interposed tissue at these two wavelengths is compared to an algorithm of oxygen saturation derived from healthy human volunteers, and a microprocessor computes the patient's SpO_2 based on this.

The phasic emission of light differentiates the light absorbance of the arterial blood from that of the light absorbance of venous blood and the surrounding tissue.

Hanning CD, Alexander-Williams JM. Fortnightly review: pulse oximetry: a practical review. BMJ. 1995;311:367–70.

Jubran A. Pulse oximetry. Intensive Care Med. 2004;30:2017–20.

Mendelson Y. Pulse oximetry: theory and applications for noninvasive monitoring. Clin Chem. 1992;38:1601.

2.9 Optical Plethysmography

2

Light transmitted through tissue is absorbed by *static elements* (muscle, bone, venous blood, and the static components of arterial blood), as well as the *pulse added volume* of arterial blood. The pulsatile arterial signal typically comprises 0.5–5 % of the total transmitted light.

The principle of optical plethysmography is made use of to display the amplitude of pulse and the heart rate. Each peak of the arterial waveform corresponds to one cardiac cycle. Occasionally a smaller secondary peak due to the venous pressure pulse can be distinguished. The phasic signal presented to the sensor, calculates the pulse amplitude according to the relative light absorbencies during systole and diastole.

Ventricular systole	Ventricular diastole
Phasic increase of blood volume in perfused organs.	Phasic decrease of blood volume in perfused organs.
Light has to travel a longer distance through the *distended* subcutaneous tissue (of the finger or ear lobe).	Light has to travel a shorter distance through the contracted subcutaneous tissue (of the finger or ear lobe).
Light transmission through the sampling site decreases.	Light transmission through the sampling site increases.

This difference is made use of to generate a waveform which is displayed on the monitor.

Mendelson Y. Pulse oximetry: theory and applications for noninvasive monitoring. Clin Chem. 1992;38:1601.

2.10   Types of Pulse Oximeters

Transmission pulse oximeters	Reflectance pulse oximeters
The conventional oximeters. A pair of light emitting diodes (LEDs) emit light through 5 to 10 mm of interposed tissue (typically a finger,toe or an earlobe,but also the bridge of nose, nares, cheek, tongue).	Photowaves from LEDs are bounced off an appropriate surface (e.g. the skull bone). This promising technology, once improved, should address several of the drawbacks in current oximeters
The change in light frequency is read out by a photodetector placed on the *opposite side* of the interposed tissue.	The reflected beam of light passes back through the tissue, (e.g. the skin of the forehead), to reach a photodetector placed *adjacent* to the LEDs.

With advancements in technology, pulse oximeters have become less expensive, smaller, lighter, and more robust. Improved algorithms now ensure fewer artefacts in measurement.

CO-oximetry
Standard pulse oximetry cannot differentiate carboxyhemoglobin from oxyhemoglobin. CO-oximeters measure absorption at several wavelengths and are primarily used to monitor SpO_2 in carboxy-hemoglobinemia (CO poisoning), and methemoglobinemia. CO-oximeters require blood sampling, though newer oximeters that pulse light at eight wavelengths are now available that reliably measure carboxyhemoglobin and methemoglobin.

Barker SJ, Curry J, Redford D, et al. Measurement of carboxyhemoglobin and methemoglobin by pulse oximetry: a human volunteer study. Anesthesiology. 2006;105:892–7.

Marr J, Abramo TJ. Monitoring in critically ill children. In: Baren JM, Rothrock SG, Brennan JA, Brown L, editors. Pediatric emergency medicine. Philadelphia: Saunders Elsevier; 2008. p. 50–2.

Tallon RW. Oximetry: state-of-the-art. Nurs Manage. 1996;27:43.

2.11   Pulse Oximetry and PaO$_2$

One of the main disadvantages of oximetry is that it monitors oxygen saturation (SpO$_2$) and not the PaO$_2$.

SpO$_2$ can miss a drop in PaO$_2$.

Major changes in PaO$_2$ on the flat upper segment of the ODC can occur without appreciable changes in SpO$_2$.

SpO$_2$ is unreliable in severe hypoxemia.

Below an SpO$_2$ of 80 %, oximetry is not dependable

SpO$_2$ can be influenced by a shift of the oxy-hemoglobin dissociation curve.	*Leftward shift of the* oxy-hemoglobin dissociation curve (as in alkalemia or hypothermia).	Hemoglobin is more saturated relative to the PaO$_2$. SpO2 can overestimate the PaO$_2$.
	Rightward shift of the oxy-hemoglobin dissociation curve (as in acidemia or fever).	Hemoglobin is less saturated relative to the *PaO$_2$. SpO$_2$ can underestimate the PaO$_2$.*

Lastly, stating the obvious, oximetry measures oxygenation but gives no information about *ventilation*; for the latter, capnography or PaCO$_2$ measurements (by arterial blood gas sampling) are required.

Ralston AC, Webb RK, Runciman WB. Potential errors in pulse oximetry. III: Effects of interference, dyes, dyshaemoglobins and other pigments. Anaesthesia 1991;46:291–295.

Stoneham MD. Uses and limitations of pulse oximetry. Br J Hosp Med. 1995;54:35.

2.12   P$_{50}$

2

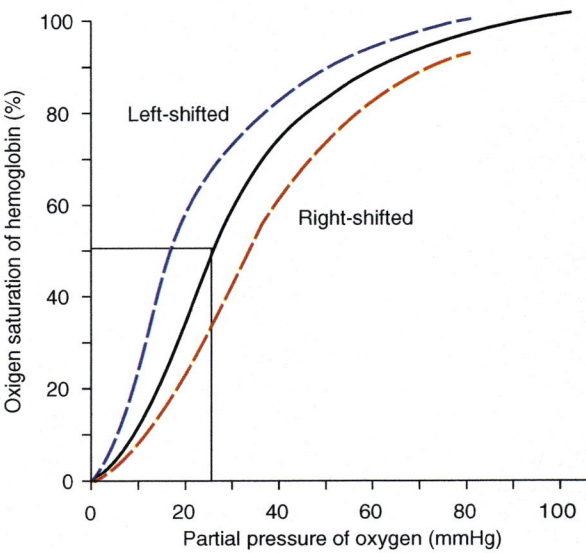

P$_{50}$

The position of the oxy-Hb dissociation curve (ODC) can be assessed from the P$_{50}$, which is the PaO$_2$ at which the Hb is 50 % saturated.

The normal P$_{50}$ is 26.6 mmHg

P$_{50}$ < 26.6 mmHg

A lower than normal P$_{50}$ means a leftward shifted ODC.

P$_{50}$ > 26.6 mmHg

A higher than normal P$_{50}$ means a rightward shifted ODC.

2.13   Shifts in the Oxy-hemoglobin Dissociation Curve

2

Leftward shift of the ODC occurs in the following conditions:	Rightward shift of the ODC occurs in the following conditions:

Alkalemia Hypothermia Abnormal hemoglobins, e.g:
    Carboxy-hemoglobin
    Met-hemoglobin
    Fetal hemoglobin
 Myxedema
 Low inorganic phosphates
 Acute pancreatitis*
	Acidemia Fever Abnormal hemoglobins, e.g.: *Hb Kansas*
	 Thyrotoxicosis
	 Raised inorganic phosphate
	 Anemia
	 Steroid therapy

Implications of a leftward shifted ODC:	**Implications of a rightward shifted ODC:**

Within the blood:
   Tighter binding of O_2 to Hb.
 At the peripheral tissues:
   With a left shifted ODC, SpO_2 is higher, but less of the O_2 (which is tightly bound to the Hb) is released to the tissues.
	Within the blood:
	   "Looser" binding of O_2 to Hb.
	 At the peripheral tissues:
	   With a right shifted ODC, although the SpO_2 is lower, more of the O_2 (which is relatively loosely bound to the Hb) is released to the tissues.

The PaO_2 is low relative to the SpO_2.	**The PaO_2 is high relative to the SpO_2.**
With a left-shifted ODC the SpO_2 may be falsely reassuring, and the PaO_2 may be lower than expected.	*The right shifted ODC facilitates oxygen delivery to the peripheraltissues.*
SpO_2 overestimates the oxygenation (i.e. PaO_2).	**SpO_2 underestimates the PaO_2.**

*Linolenic acid, Linoleic acid and Oleic acid, the fatty acids released into the circulation as a result of pancreatic cell destruction, bind to hemoglobin and increase its affinity for O_2.

Greenberg AG, Terlizzi L, Peskin G. Oxyhemoglobin affinity in acute pancreatitis. J Surg Res. 1977;22:561–5.

2.14   Oxygen Saturation (SpO_2) in Anemia and Skin Pigmentation

Anemia unless it is very severe (Hb < 5 g/dl) does not influence the SpO_2.

Since SpO_2 is expressed as a percentage of the available binding sites for O_2, anemia can critically affect the O_2 content of the blood (CaO_2), but has virtually no impact on SpO_2.

The amount of Hb in the blood determines the O_2 content of the blood, not the SpO_2.

The colour of the interposed tissue can influence the SpO_2.

Skin pigmentation	Hyper-bilirubin-emia	Nail polish	
Minor and inconsistent effect on SpO_2. However some studies have shown that racial pigmentation may cause as much as 4 % difference in measured SpO_2.	Minimal effect on SpO_2.	**Red nail polish** May have a trivial effect on SpO_2.	**Other shades of nail polish** May produce a spurious fall in SpO_2 of as much as 3–6 %.

Schnapp LM, Cohen NH. Pulse oximetry: uses and abuses. Chest. 1990;98:1244.

2.15 Oxygen Saturation (SpO$_2$) in Abnormal Forms of Hemoglobin

Abnormal forms of hemoglobin can have very different absorption spectra, and oximetric readings (SpO$_2$) can overestimate the true oxygen saturation of Hb (see Sect. 2.20)

CO-Hb* *SpO$_2$ over-estimates SaO$_2$*	CO-Hb has an almost identical absorption spectrum (660 ηm) to oxy-Hb.	Because the oximeter interprets CO-Hb as normal Hb, normal SpO$_2$ can be displayed even in severe hypoxia. Diagnosis is by CO-oximetry (Sect. 2.19).
Met-Hb** *SpO$_2$ over-estimates SaO$_2$*	Met-Hb absorbs light at both wavelengths 660 ηm and 940 ηm) that standard oximeters emit. Because of this property, Met-Hb has a complex effect on SpO$_2$.	At low levels of Met-Hb, SaO$_2$ overestimates the SpO$_2$. When Met-Hb levels increase to over 30 %, SpO$_2$ tends to drift towards 85 %, which is a gross overestimation of SaO$_2$. Presumptive diagnosis is by CO-oximetry; it is confirmed by the Evelyn-Malloy method (Sect. 2.26 and 2.27).
Hb-S*** *Variably affects SpO$_2$*	Hb-S has a similar absorption spectrum to oxy-Hb.	Hb-S can lead to spuriously high or low SpO$_2$ values.
Fetal Hb	Has no special impact on SpO$_2$	

*Carboxy-hemoglobin **Met-hemoglobin *** in Sickle-cell disease

Barker SJ, Curry J, Redford D, et al. Measurement of carboxyhemoglobin and methemoglobin by pulse oximetry: a human volunteer study. Anesthesiology. 2006;105:892–7.

Eisenkraft JI, Pulse oximeter desaturation due to methemoglobinemia. Anesthesiology. 1988;68:279.

Ernst A, Zibrak JD. Carbon monoxide poisoning. New Engl J Med. 1998;339:1603–8.

Evelyn K, Malloy H. Microdetermination of oxyhemoglobin, methemoglobin, and sulfhemoglobin in a single sample of blood. J Biol Chem. 1938;126:655.

Ortiz FO, Aldrich TK, Nagel RL, Benjamin LJ. Accuracy of pulse oximetry in sickle cell disease. Am J Respir Crit Care Med. 1999;159:447.

2.16   Mechanisms of Hypoxemia in Methemoglobinemia

2

Normal hemoglobin	Methemoglobin
Normal hemoglobin carries its iron as ferrous ions. Hb is capable of binding O_2 provided the ferrous iron remains in its reduced state. The special configuration of the hemoglobin chains appears to protect the ferrous ions from oxidation to the ferric state. **Pulmonary capillaries** In the pulmonary capillaries each ferrous iron moiety binds an O_2 atom, in the process briefly donating an electron to the latter. **Tissue capillaries** At the tissue capillary level the O_2 atom cleaves away from the Hb molecule, in the process reacquiring its electron. The reduction of the iron back to its ferrous form makes it free to bind and transport O_2 again.	**Met-Hb carries its iron as ferric ions.** Met-Hb, as opposed to deoxy-Hb carries its iron in the ferric form, in which state it is unable to bind O_2. That amount of Hb that exists as Met-Hb cannot participate in O_2 transport. Also, the ferrous iron that is present in the adjacent hemoglobin chains binds more strongly to O_2 than usual. The oxygen dissociation curve is shifted to the left leaving little O_2 for the tissues.

Methemoglobin has peak absorbance at 631 ηm. CO-oximeters use a fixed wavelength to screen for methemoglobin: all readings in the 630 ηm range are reported as methemoglobin. Several pigments (including sulfhemoglobin and methylene blue) can evoke false positive results.

Curry S. Methemoglobinemia. Ann Emerg Med. 1982;11:214–21.

Wright RO, Lewander WJ, Woolf AD. Methemoglobinemia: etiology, pharmacology, and clinical management. Ann Emerg Med. 1999;34:646–56.

2.17   Methemoglobinemias: Classification

2

Methemoglobinemias can be classified into the hereditary methemoglobinemias and the acquired methemoglobinemias.

The acquired methemoglobinemias are due to extrinsic agents, *which result in increased formation of Met-Hb.*	In the **hereditary methemoglobinemias,** faulty pathways result in *decreased reduction of Met-Hb, which consequently accumulates.*	
e.g.: • p-Amino salicylic acid • Aniline dyes • Benzene derivatives • Clofazimine • Chlorates • Chloroquine • Dapsone • Local anesthetic agents • Metoclopramide • Nitrites (eg Amyl nitrite, Nitroglycerin) • Nitric oxide • Phenacetin • Primaquine • Sulfonamides	**Cytochrome b5 reductase deficiency:** Normally about 0.5–3 % of Hb is converted to Met-Hb daily by auto-oxidation. Some of this Met-Hb gets reduced back Hb (by a NADH dependent, cytochrome b5 reductase catalysed reaction 0. As a result, Met-Hb comprises about 1 % of total Hb in the blood. Cytochrome b5 reductase deficiency can result in increased methemoglobin levels.	**Hemoglobin-M disease:** As a result of a mutation in the alpha or beta globin chain, tyrosine replaces one of the histidine residues. Ferric phenolate complex formed: Fe^{+++} cannot be effectively reduced to the ferrous state. Persistent lifelong methemoglobinemia occurs.

Curry S. Methemoglobinemia. Ann Emerg Med. 1982;11:214–21.

Jaffe ER. Enzymopenic hereditary methemoglobinemia: a clinical/biochemical classification. Blood Cells. 1986;12:81–90.

Prchal JT. Clinical features, diagnosis and treatment of methemoglobinemia. In: Basow DS, editors. UpToDate. Waltham: UpToDate; 2012. Last updated 22 Mar 2012. Last accessed 13 May 2012.

2.18   Sulfhemoglobinemia

STEP 1: Oxidation of Hb to methemoglobin

First, the oxidation of the ferrous to ferric iron results in the formation of methemoglobin.

STEP 2: Formation of sulfhemoglobin

Next, the exposure to specific agents results in covalent binding of the sulfur atom to heme, resulting in the formation of sulfhemoglobin.

Similarities with methemoglobinemia

Sulfhemoglobin, like methemoglobin, can neither transport O_2 nor CO_2.

Differences with methemoglobinemia
Right shift of ODC
Unlike Met-Hb, Sulf-Hb causes a right shift of ODC and so relatively more oxygen is released to the tissues.

Severity of hypoxia
Hypoxia in sulfhemoglobinemia is not as severe as that in methemoglobinemia.

Sulfhemoglobinemia is irreversible
Unlike methemoglobinemia, sulfhemoglobinemia is irreversible.

Oximeters that measure Met-Hb can erroneously read Sulf-Hb as Met-Hb

---

Park CM, Nagel RL. Sulfhemoglobinemia. N Engl J Med. 1984;310:1579–84.

2.19   Carbon Monoxide (CO) Poisoning

2

The incomplete combustion of hydrocarbons leads to the formation of CO, a colour-less, odourless gas. Normally, the levels of carboxy-hemoglobin (CO-Hb) are <3 % of total Hb in the urban population; smokers have a CO-Hb level of 5–10 % of total Hb in their blood. At levels above 50 %, CO-Hb is capable of causing death.

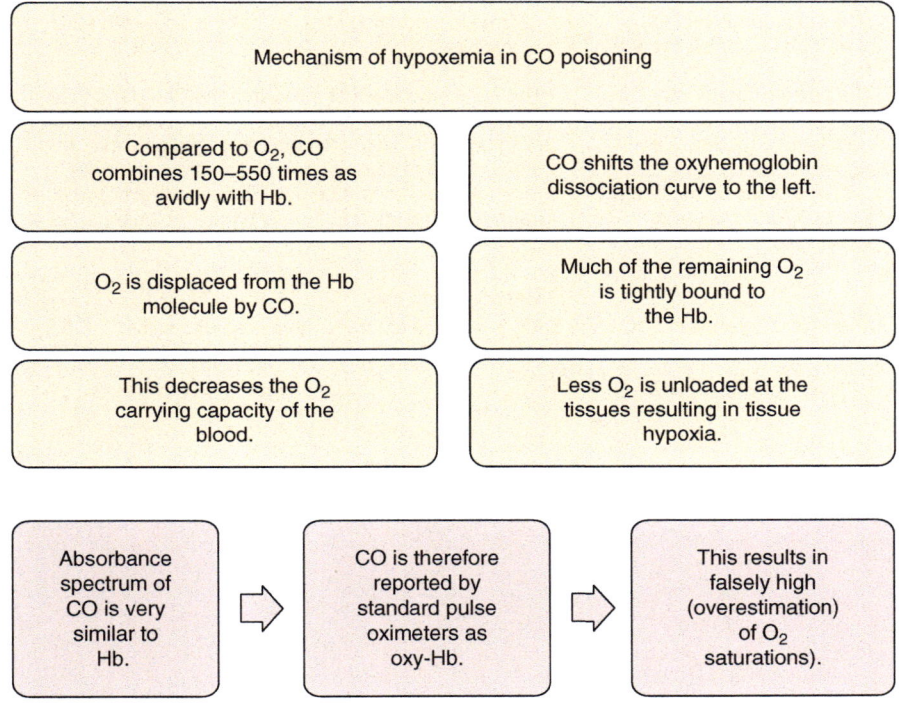

CO-oximetry (multi-wavelength spectrophotometry that separately measures CO-Hb, Oxy-Hb, and reduced Hb) reliably measures CO levels and should be used when CO poisoning is suspected (Sect. 2.10).

Caughey WS. Carbon monoxide bonding in hemeproteins. Ann N Y Acad Sci. 1970;174:148.
Weaver LK. Carbon monoxide poisoning. Crit Care Clin. 1999;15:297.

2.20   Saturation Gap

The O_2 analyses by the pulse oximeter and the ABG are based upon the premise that only two forms of Hb are possible: Oxyhemoglobin and deoxyhemoglobin; and that no abnormal forms of hemoglobin are present.

***SpO$_2$** (low)*	***SaO$_2$** (normal)*
The Hb saturation of O_2 as measured by pulse oximetry.	The Hb saturation of O_2 as calculated by the ABG machine.
The pulse oximeter measures light absorbance at two wavelengths (2.08). With significant levels of methemoglobin in the blood, the SpO$_2$ drifts towards 85 % (2.16).	The ABG machine first measures the PaO$_2$ and then calculates the expected SaO$_2$ from this, based on the position of the oxyhemoglobin dissociation curve. In the absence of cardiopulmonary disease, the SaO$_2$ (not being dependent on oxy-Hb concentration) will be normal even though abnormal hemoglobins be present.

The saturation gap

When the difference in SaO$_2$ and SpO$_2$ is >5 %, a saturation gap is said to exist.
A saturation gap is a clue to significant levels of certain abnormal hemoglobins in the blood (Sect. 2.15, 2.16, 2.17, 2.18 and 2.19).

Eisenkraft JI. Pulse oximeter desaturation due to methemoglobinemia. Anesthesiology. 1988;68:279.

Haymond S, Cariappa R, Eby CS, Scott MG. Laboratory assessment of oxygenation in methemoglobinemia. Clin Chem. 2005;51(2):434–44.

Mokhlesi B, Leiken JB, Murray P, Corbridge TC. Adult toxicology in critical care, part I: general approach to the intoxicated patient. Chest. 2003;123:577–92.

Oesenberg B. Pulse oximetry in methaemoglobinemia. Anaesthesia. 1990;45:56.

2.21   Sources of Error While Measuring SpO$_2$

Time lag	*Output stabilization:* There is often a time lag between a change in O$_2$ saturation and its detection by the oximeter. The signal averaging by the oximeter may take several seconds. This can be disadvantageous in a rapidly changing clinical situation. Modern pulse oximeters take less than a minute for output stabilisation to occur. Subsequent SpO$_2$ changes usually take less than ten seconds to register. Response time: toe>finger>earlobe.
Weak signal	*Hypoperfusion of the interposed part: SpO$_2$ falsely low* Vasoconstriction BP < 80 mmHg Inflation of a BP cuff Edema of an extremity
	Noise amplification: When the pulse is weak, the pulse oximeter boosts its amplitude. In doing so it may amplify the background noise and lead to errors. Most current devices warn of weak pulse strength may simply not display the saturation.
Proximity to instruments	MRI scanners Cell-phones Electrical interference Power outlets and cords, cardiac monitors, cautery devices etc.
Motion artifact	Shivering Convulsions Movement
Arrythmias	Irregular rhythms such as atrial fibrillation can unpredictably affect displayed values.
Optical issues	*Optical shunt: underestimation of the SpO$_2$* Light from the photodiode reaches the photodetector without passing through the interposed part (penumbra effect). A calculated SpO$_2$ (usually in the low eighties) will result in underestimation of the actual SpO$_2$. *Light interference: underestimation of the SpO$_2$* Light interference may occur by extraneous light directly impinging on the photodetector especially if the probe is too large or improperly placed. Ambient light, direct sunlight, fluorescent, infrared, and xenon lamps may cause interference. The calculated SpO$_2$ tends towards 85 % and is therefore underestimated. Execptionally (strong ambient light, completely displaced probe), the SpO$_2$ may be falsely high.

To avoid errors, the amplitude of the pulse waveform should be routinely checked. In the presence of a satisfactory waveform with an observable dicrotic notch, the SpO$_2$ readings are likely to be correct. A close agreement between the displayed pulse rate on the oximeter and the manually counted pulse rate suggests that the SpO$_2$ reading is likely to be correct. When the pulse signal is strong, pulse oximeters are accurate provided saturations range above 80 %. At lower saturations however, they lose some of their reliability. When the stroke output fluctuates synchronously with the respiratory cycle (such as in a ventilated patient who develops auto-PEEP), the tracing will oscillate noticeably about the baseline.

Rarely, pulse oximetry has been associated with complications. Prolonged use on hypoperfused digits can potentially cause digital injury. Metal components of oximeter probes will heat up in strong electromagnetic fields, and the use of non-MRI compatible oximeter probes during MRI scanning has been associated with thermal injury.

Cannesson M, Attof Y, Rosamel P, et al. Respiratory variations in pulse oximetry plethysmographic waveform amplitude to predict fluid responsiveness in the operating room. Anesthesiology. 2007;44(4):273–9.

Costarino AT, Davis DA, Keon TP. Falsely normal saturation reading with the pulse oximeter. Anesthesiology. 1987;67:830–1.

Dempsey MF, Condon B. Thermal injuries associated with MRI. Clin Radiol 2001;56:457–65.

Gehring H, Hornberger C, Matz H, et al. The effects of motion artifact and low perfusion on the performance of a new generation of pulse oximeters in volunteers undergoing hypoxemia. Respir Care. 2002;47:48.

Hinkelbein J, Genzwuerker HV, Fielder F. Detection of a systolic pressure threshold for reliable readings in pulse oximetry. Resuscitation. 2005;64:315.

Kelleher JF, Ruff RH. The penumbra effect: vasomotion–dependent pulse oximeter artifact due to probe malposition. Anesthesiology. 1989;71:787–91.

Lee WW, Mayberry K, Crapo R, Jensen RL. The accuracy of pulse oximetry in the emergency department. Am J Emerg Med. 2000;18:427.

Poets CF, Seidenberg J, von der Hardt H. Failure of a pulse oximeter to detect sensor displacement. Lancet. 1993;341:244.

Ralston AC, Webb RK, Runciman WB. Potential errors in pulse oximetry. III: Effects of interference, dyes, dyshaemoglobins and other pigments. Anaesthesia 1991;46:291–295.

Van de Louw A, Cracco C, Cerf C, et al. Accuracy of pulse oximetry in the intensive care unit. Intensive Care Med. 2001;27:1606.

Wille J, Braams R, van Haren WH, et al. Pulse oximeter–induced digital injury: frequency rate and possible causative factors. Crit Care Med. 2000;28:3555–7.

2.22   Point of Care (POC) Cartridges

Point of Care (POC) cartridges are now in use for the bedside measurement of the pH, PaCO$_2$ and PaO$_2$.

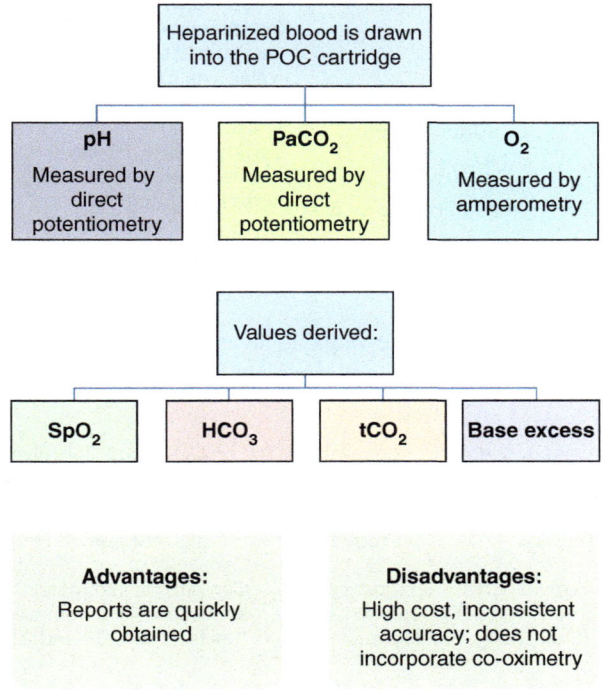

Canham EM. Interpretation of arterial blood gases. In: Parsons PE, Weiner-Kronish JP, editors. Critical care secrets. 3rd ed. Philadelphia: Hanley and Belfus, Inc, 2003; p. 21–4.

2.23   Capnography and Capnometry

Capnography	Capnometry
Capnography is the real time monitoring of the exhaled CO_2 over time (or sometimes, over volume): it is displayed as a waveform.	Capnometry is the non-invasive measurement of exhaled CO_2, which is displayed as an end expiratory (end-tidal) value. The inspiratory and expiratory levels of CO_2 are shown as a partial pressure or percentage on a digital or analog display. However, the terms capnography and capnometry are often used interchangeably.

Time Capnography:	Volume Capnography:
The CO_2 levels displayed against *time* on the x axis.	The CO_2 levels displayed against *expired volume* on the x axis.

Waveform analysis can provide valuable information regarding the adequacy of gas sampling, and leaks in tubing, and can identify certain prevailing disorders.

Capnograph waveform analysis provides information on CO_2 production, alveolar ventilation, perfusion, breathing pattern, status of the ventilator circuit and endotracheal tube position.

Height (E_tCO_2)	Frequency	Shape	Height
E_tCO_2 is the maximum partial pressure of CO_2 achieved at end-exhalation (Sect. 2.24).	Frequency represents the respiratory rate.	Can provide information about specific abnormalities (Sects. 2.35, 2.36 and 2.37).	See (Sect. 2.35)

*CO_2 measurements techniques use Raman spectrography, mass spectrography, photoacoustic spectrography and chemical colorimetric analysis and infrared spectrography. The last is the most widely used. Single-use qualitative colorimetric end-tidal CO_2 detectors use indicator discs that change color when the CO_2 concentration of exhaled gas exceeds 2 %: from purple ($EtCO_2 < 3$ mmHg) to yellow ($EtCO_2 > 15$ mmHg).

Sullivan KJ, Kissoon N, Goodwin SR. End–tidal carbon dioxide monitoring in pediatric emergencies. Pediatr Emerg Care. 2005;21(5):327–32.

2.24   The Capnographic Waveform

The capnographic wave form is divided into six distinct parts.

A–B: dead-space exhalation	The first part of exhalation contains air from the proximal airway (the conductive zone of the lung).	This air is devoid of CO_2, (provided there is no rebreathing) and so the CO_2 waveform is a flat line that hugs the baseline.
B: the onset of alveolar exhalation	Alveolar air contains CO_2.	As alveolar air begins to arrive at the sampling site, the capnograph shows a sudden upturn.
B–C: the continuance of alveolar exhalation	The CO_2 rises rapidly as alveolar gas mixed with dead-space gas arrives at the sensor.	The capnograph shows a steep upslope.
C–D: the alveolar plateau	Most of the gas received at the sensor is now alveolar gas.	The gradually upsloping plateau represents the constant emptying of viable alveoli.
D: End-tidal CO_2 (E_tCO_2)	The peak at the end of the plateau represents the averaging of alveolar CO_2 levels.	The peak represents the end-tidal CO_2.
D–E: inspiratory washout	The graph then falls rapidly to the baseline.	The nadir represents the negligible CO_2 (0.003 % or 0.02 mmHg) that reaches the alveoli from the ambient air.

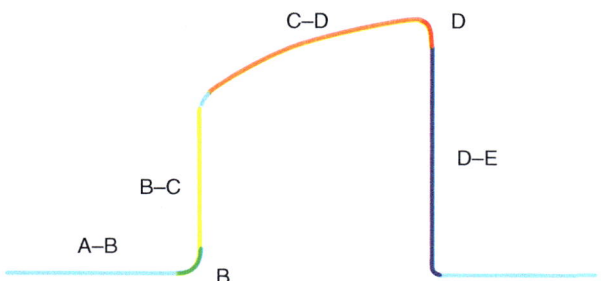

Stock MC. Capnography for adults. Crit Care Clinics. 1995;11:219.

2.25   Main-Stream and Side-Stream Capnometers

Mainstream capnometers	Side-stream capnometers
A CO_2 sensor (infrared detector) mounted on a cuvette (T- adapter) is interposed between the ET and the patient-circuit. CO_2 analysis is performed within the airway, obviating the need for need for gas sampling	A relatively long sampling tube connected to the piece draws away the gas sample to a CO_2 sensor located in a central unit. The sampling flow rate can be as high as 150 ml/min. This can result in substantial deformation of the waveform when low tidal volumes are used as in neonates and infants.
There is no sampling tube. Sensor windows are prone to clogging by secretions, aerosols or water droplets.	Sampling tube prone to becoming obstructed as secretion can be sucked in by the rapid aspiration rate. Leakages from the circuit are possible (Sect. 2.27)
No time lag owing to the centrally located processor.	Time lag in display (CO_2 flight time) owing to the distance of the sensor from the airway.
Unaffected by changes in water vapour pressure. The temperature within is maintained at around 39°C to prevent condensation (which can spuriously elevate E_tCO_2).	Affected by changes in water vapour pressure. By slightly modifying the standard nasal cannulae, it is possible to make fairly precise measurements even in patients breathing supplemental oxygen through nasal cannulae.
Cannot be used in the absence of an artificial airway.	Since exhaled gas is sampled from the nasal cavity using nasal adaptors, measurement is possible in the absence of an artificial airway.
Difficult to use in patients undergoing prone ventilation.	Relatively easy to connect in unusual positions (such as prone position).
Sterilization is difficult.	Easy to sterilize.
Can increase circuit dead-space & so elevate PaCO$_2$	Side stream capnometers using micro-stream technology have been developed. Using sampling flow rates of as low as 50 ml/min**. The emitted wavelength is within a narrower IR band (4.2–4.35 µm) which more closely matches the absorption spectrum for CO_2.

*Burns may occur if the heated sensing head lies in contact with the patient's skin.
**The rate of gas sampling ranges from 50 to 2,000 ml/min (usually 50–200 ml/min). When the sampling flow rate exceeds the expired gas flow, contamination from the base gas flow source is inevitable.

Kalenda Z. Mastering infrared capnography. Utrecht, The Netherlands: Kerckebosch-Zeist, 1989, p101.

Moon RE, Camporesi EM. Respiratory monitoring. In: Miller RD, editor. Miller's anesthesia. 6th ed. Philadelphia: Elsevier/Churchill Livingstone; 2005.

2.26 $P_{Et}CO_2$ (E_tCO_2): A Surrogate for $PaCO_2$

2

CO_2 diffuses rapidly across all biological membranes including the alveolo-capillary membrane. Arterial CO_2 ($PaCO_2$) equilibrates rapidly with alveolar CO_2 ($PACO_2$), and is effectively identical with it. $P_{Et}CO_2$ offers a non-invasive means of monitoring $PaCO_2$, given that:

In health:	In disease:
The value of $P_{Et}CO_2$ is close to the value of $PACO_2$; and therefore to that of $PaCO_2$. $PaCO_2$ and $PACO_2$ differ by such a small amount (generally < 5 mm) such as usually makes no clinical difference. The trends in $P_{Et}CO_2$ closely match the trends in $PaCO_2$.	In disease, physiological dead-space is often increased because of patent but under-perfused alveoli. Due to the lack of an effective pulmonary circulation CO_2 cannot effectively diffuse into alveoli. Under such circumstances, $PaCO_2$ can substantially exceed $P_{Et}CO_2$. In spite of this, in the absence of major *changes* in dead-space ventilation, the $P_{Et}CO_2$ trends still match those of $PaCO_2$.

CO_2 values cannot be used as an absolute surrogate for $PaCO_2$. However the E_tCO_2 may be expected to *parallel* the changes in $PaCO_2$ (i.e, the [A-a]CO_2 gradient remains constant) provided that:

Stable cardiac condition	Stable pulmonary condition	Stable body temperature

Fletcher R, Jonson B. Deadspace and the single breath test for carbon dioxide during anaesthesia and artificial ventilation. Br J Anaeasth. 1984;56:109–19.

Nunn JF, Hill DW. Respiratory dead space and arterial to end-tidal CO_2 tension difference in anesthetized man. J Appl Physiol. 1960;15:383–9.

Shankar KB, Moseley H, Kumar Y, Vemula V. Arterial to end-tidal carbon dioxide tension difference during cesarean section anaesthesia. Anaesthesia. 1986;41:698–702.

2.27   Factors Affecting $P_{Et}CO_2$

Factors that increase $P_{Et}CO_2$	Factors that decrease $P_{Et}CO_2$
Increase in CO_2 production*: Fever, shivering, convulsions; infusion of $NaHCO_3$, blood, glucose or parenteral nutrients Release of a tourniquet CO_2 insufflation or embolism	**Decreased CO_2 production:** Hypothermia
Increase in pulmonary perfusion: Increase in cardiac output Increase in blood pressure	**Decrease in pulmonary perfusion:** Decreased cardiac output Fall in BP, hypovolemia Pulmonary embolism Wedged PA catheter
Decrease in alveolar ventilation: Hypoventilation (see Sect. 1.35)	**Increase in alveolar ventilation** Hyperventilation
Airway related problems Bronchial intubation Partial airway obstruction	**Airway related problems** Accidental extubation Partial or complete airway obstruction Apnea
Machine-related factors: CO_2 scrubber used up Insufficient inflow of fresh gas Leaks in circuit Malfunctioning ventilator valves	**Machine-related factors:** Circuit disconnection Leakage of gas during sampling: gas pump, flow regulator, sampling system (connector to the sampling port, water trap) Malfunction of ventilator

*Unlike in paralyzed mechanically ventilated patients, an increase in CO_2 production will not lead to a rise in $P_{Et}CO_2$ in spontaneously breathing individuals (owing to the reflex hyperventilation that a high CO_2 level evokes in these persons).

(Modified from: Kodali BS. Factors influencing $P_{Et}CO_2$. 2007. Welcome to capnography.com. Last accessed 6 June 2012.)

Shankar KB, Moseley H, Kumar AY, Delph Y. Capnometry and anaesthesia. Review article. Can J Anaesth. 1992;39(6):617–32.

2.28   Causes of Increased PaCO$_2$-P$_{Et}$CO$_2$ Difference

2

> **Increased PaCO$_2$-P$_{Et}$CO$_2$ difference, (a-A)CO$_2$**
> Increased a-ACO$_2$ difference implies increased dead-space.
> Very rarely is a sharp increase in CO$_2$ production
> responsible for a widened a-ACO$_2$.

Increased physiological dead-space:

Decreased pulmonary perfusion

Global decrease in pulmonary perfusion

Decrease in LV output

Regional decrease in pulmonary perfusion

Pulmonary embolism

Increased CO$_2$ production

As a cause of increased A-aCO$_2$, increased PaCO$_2$ is distinctly uncommon. In such cases, the increase in A-aO$_2$ is usually transient.

Phan CQ, Tremper KK, Lee SE, Barker SJ. Noninvasive monitoring of carbon dioxide: a comparison of the partial pressure of transcutaneous and end-tidal carbon dioxide with the partial pressure of arterial carbon dioxide. J Clin Monit. 1987;3:149–54.

2.29   Bohr's Equation

2

It is possible to estimate the dead space, utilizing Bohr's equation.

All the exhaled CO_2 comes from the alveolar gas. None of the exhaled CO_2 comes from the dead-space air.
Therefore,

$$VT = VA + VD$$

Or, tidal volume (VT) = Alveolar gas volume (VA) + dead-space gas (VD)
Rearranging,

$$VA = VT–VD ...(Eq 2.1)$$

$$VT \times FECO_2 = VA \times FACO_2 ...(Eq 2.2)$$

Where,
VT = tidal volume
$FECO_2$ = Fractional concentration of CO_2 in exhaled gas
VA = Alveolar gas volume
$FACO_2$ = Fractional concentration of CO_2 in alveolar gas

Substituting the value of VA (Eq 2.1) within Eq 2.2
$$VT \times FECO_2 = (VT–VD) \times FACO_2$$
Therefore,
$$VD/VT = (FACO_2–FECO_2) / FACO_2$$

Since the partial pressure of a gas is proportional to its concentration, the equation can be rewritten as "Bohr's equation":

$$VD/VT = (PACO_2 – PECO_2)/PACO_2$$

And since the PCO_2 of alveolar gas ($PACO_2$) very nearly equals the PCO_2 of arterial gas ($PaCO_2$),

$$VD/VT = (PaCO_2 – PECO_2)/PaCO_2$$

Thus, by simultaneously measuring the end-expiratory CO_2 ($P_{Et}CO_2$) and the $PaCO_2$, the dead-space to tidal volume ratio can be calculated (see Sect. 2.30).

Criner GJ, D'Alonzo G, editors. Pulmonary pathophysiology. Lyndell: Fence Creek Publishing Co.; 1998.

Shankar KB, Moseley H, Kumar AY, Delph Y. Capnometry and anaesthesia. Review article. Can J Anaesth. 1992;39(6):617-32.

2.30   Application of Bohr's Equation

2

Consider the following data in a patient:

Tidal volume (VT) = 500 mL
Breaths per minute (f) = 12
Minute ventilation = 6,000
mL/min
$PaCO_2$ = 40 mmHg
E_tCO_2 = 30 mmHg

$VD/VT = (PaCO_2–PECO_2)/PaCO_2$
$VD/VT = (40–30)/40$
$VD/VT = 10/40 = 0.25$
(The normal VD/VT is 0.20–0.35 at
rest)

With a VD/VT of 0.25 and a tidal
volume of 500 mL,
$VD = 0.25 \times 500 = 125$ mL
We know that alveolar ventilation
$= (VT–VD) \times f$
Alveolar ventilation = $(500 – 125) \times$
$12 = 4,500$ mL

Criner GJ, D'Alonzo G, editors. Pulmonary pathophysiology. Lyndell: Fence Creek Publishing Co.; 1998.

2.31   Variations in E_tCO_2

Discrepancy between the $PaCO_2$ and the $P_{Et}CO_2$ can occur when there is an increase in the dead-space, or if a significant V/Q mismatch occurs. The impact of pulmonary disease on $P_{Et}CO_2$ is unpredictable and widening of the gradient often occurs.

On rare occasions, when large tidal volumes are used to inflate lungs with low-V/Q ratios, the $P_{Et}CO_2$ may actually exceed the $PaCO_2$

Since CO_2 is an easily diffusible gas with respect to biological membranes, the drop in the end-tidal CO_2 tension relative to arterial CO_2 is only about 2–5 mmHg. However, this is at best a rough approximation and in disease the end-tidal CO_2 may be prone to substantial variation.

High concentrations of either oxygen or nitrous oxide may cause variations in the capnogram as both these gases have similar infrared spectra to CO_2 and correction factors should be applied when mixtures of these gases are breathed.

Thus, in health, trends in arterial CO_2 are matched by the end-tidal CO_2. With unstable or evolving lung pathology, the end-tidal CO_2 may neither reflect nor parallel changes in $PaCO_2$.

Moorthy SS, Losasso AM, Wilcox J. End-tidal PCO_2 greater than $PaCO_2$. Chest. 1984;12:534.

2.32 False-Positive and False-Negative Capnography

FALSE NEGATIVE (a flat wave form in spite of a properly sited endotracheal tube)	
Cardiac arrest	The sluggish pulmonary blood flow delivers little CO_2 to the alveoli for excretion.
Large air leak (e.g. ruptured ET cuff)	A large amount of atmospheric air dilutes the exhaled air the CO_2-concentration of which resultantly falls.
An obstructed ET tube	CO_2 from the exhaled air has no access to the capnograph sensor.

FALSE POSITIVE (CO_2 detected on the capnograph in spite of a improperly sited endotracheal)	
Endotracheal tip resides with in the pharynx	In spite of this effective (or partially compromised) ventilation may still be possible.
Aggressive 'bagging'	Aggressive bag-and-mask ventilation has resulted in gastric distension with CO_2 containing air.
Carbonated bevereges	In animal studies, ingestion of carbonated beverages has also resulted in false positive capnographic measurements.

When capnography is false positive, the E_tCO_2 values will inevitably decline over successive breaths. It has therefore been suggested that E_tCO_2 levels be closely monitored for a minimum of six successive breaths.

The shape of the capnograph remains remarkably similar in all healthy humans. This of course means that any deviation from the typical shape must be inquired into (see following sections).

Hasan A. Esophageal intubation. In: Understanding Mechanical Ventilation: a Practical Handbook. London: Springer; 2010. p.183, 309–10.

Puntervoll SA, Soreide E, Jacewicz W, et al. Rapid detection of oesophageal intubation: take care when using colorimetric capnometry. Acta Anaesthesiol Scand. 2002;46(4):455–7.

Qureshi S, Park K, Sturmann K, et al. The effect of carbonated beverages on colorimetric end–tidal CO(2) determination. Acad Emerg Med. 2000;7(10):1169.

2.33   Capnography and Cardiac Output

2

When alveolar ventilation is constant, the $P_{Et}CO_2$ reflects pulmonary perfusion, which itself is dependent upon the cardiac output.

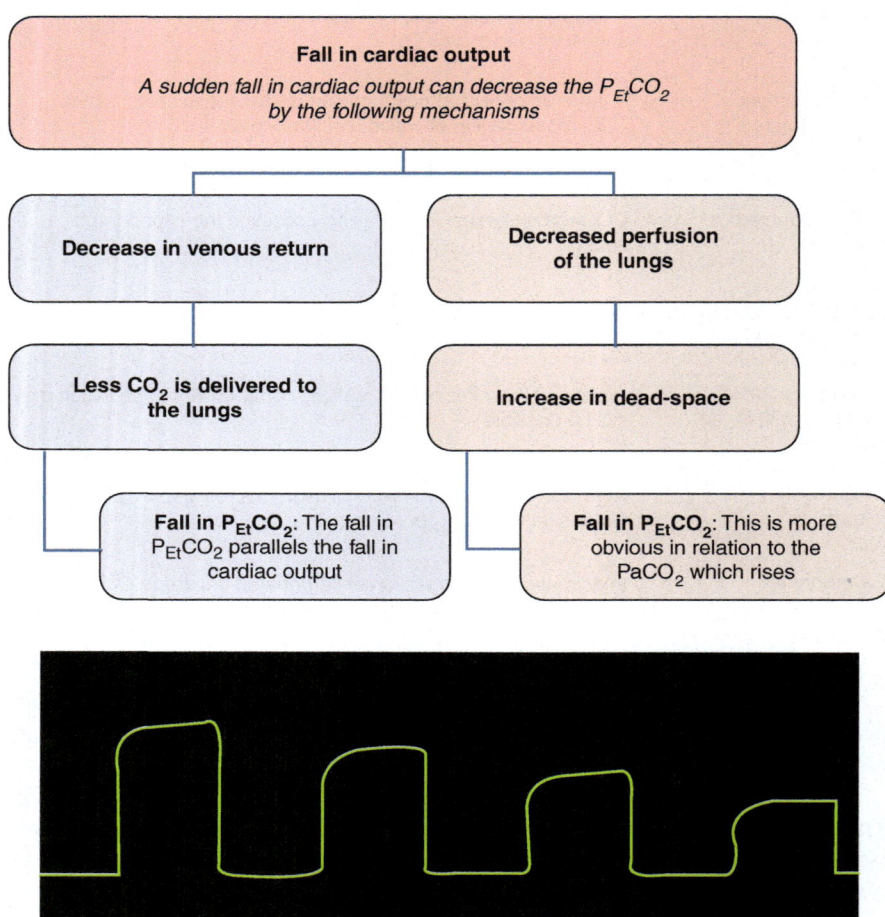

Fall in cardiac output
A sudden fall in cardiac output can decrease the $P_{Et}CO_2$ by the following mechanisms

Decrease in venous return

Decreased perfusion of the lungs

Less CO_2 is delivered to the lungs

Increase in dead-space

Fall in $P_{Et}CO_2$: The fall in $P_{Et}CO_2$ parallels the fall in cardiac output

Fall in $P_{Et}CO_2$: This is more obvious in relation to the $PaCO_2$ which rises

Real-time capnograph showing fall in cardiac output due to cardiac arrest

Isserles S, Breen PH. Can changes in end-tidal PCO_2 measure changes in cardiac output? Anesth Analg. 1991;73:808.

Shibutani K, Shirasaki S, Braaz T, et al. Changes in cardiac output affect $P_{Et}CO_2$, CO_2 transport, and O2 uptake during unsteady state in humans. J Clin Monit. 1992;8:175–6.

2.34   Capnography as a Guide to Successful Resuscitation

Using capnography, it is possible to differentiate *asphyxic cardiac arrest* (very high $P_{Et}CO_2$) from *primary cardiac arrest* (increase in $P_{Et}CO_2$ is not as high). $P_{Et}CO_2$ can provide a valuable guide to CPR.

Successful CPR	CPR resumption	CPR termination
A sudden rise in $P_{Et}CO_2$ is often the earliest indicator of the revival of the hemodynamics. It is more sensitive than the ECG, pulse, or blood pressure, and is unaffected by the artefacts produced by chest compression. The transient rise in $P_{Et}CO_2$ reflects the elimination of the CO_2 built up within tissues.	Conversely, a drop in $P_{Et}CO_2$ in apatient who has just been successfully revived may indicate the need for resumption of CPR.	In a patient with pulseless electrical activity, the $P_{Et}CO_2$ measured at 20 min after the commencement of CPR can provide a valuable guide of outcome.

$P_{Et}CO_2$ after 20 min CPR: <10 mmHg Further continuation of CPR is unlikely to be fruitful*.	$P_{Et}CO_2$ after 20 min CPR: >18 mmHg Heralds a successful out come to the CPR*.

*No specific number can assigned as a cut off value in distinguishing survivors from non-survivors: it is believed that the chances for survival increase by 16 % for every 1 mmHg that the $P_{Et}CO_2$ rises.

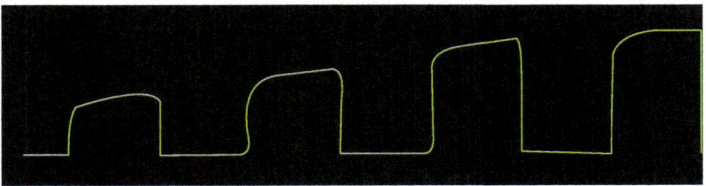

The return of spontaneous circulation following successful CPR

Callaham M, Barton C. Prediction of outcome of cardiopulmonary resuscitation from end-tidal carbon dioxide concentration. Crit Care Med. 1990;18:358.

Falk JL, Rackow ED, Weil MH. End-tidal carbon dioxide concentration during cardiopulmonary resuscitation. N Engl J Med. 1988;318(10):607–11.

Grmec S, Klemen P. Does the end-tidal carbon dioxide ($ETCO_2$) concentration have prognostic value during out-of-hospital cardiac arrest? J Emerg Med. 2001;8:263–9.

Sanders AB, Kern KB, Otto CW, et al. End-tidal carbon dioxide monitoring during cardiopulmonary resuscitation: a prognostic indicator for survival. JAMA. 1989;262:1347–51.

2.35   Capnography in Respiratory Disease

Pulse oximetry which measures *oxygenation* cannot serve as a replacement for capnography, which monitors *ventilation*. Capnography will diagnose hypoventilation long before the latter results in hypoxia, and this is especially the case in patients on supplemental oxygen. In *hypoventilation,* tall (high $P_{Et}CO_2$) low-frequency waves are manifest with a well-defined alveolar plateau (a similar waveform can occur when the dead space is increased). In *hyperventilation,* short (low $P_{Et}CO_2$) high-frequency waves with a well-defined alveolar plateau are seen.

Hypoventilation	**Hypoventilation**
The capnograph shows:	The capnograph shows:
slow respiratory rate (low frequency)	High respiratory rate (low frequency)
High CO_2 levels (tall waves)	Low CO_2 levels (relatively short waves)

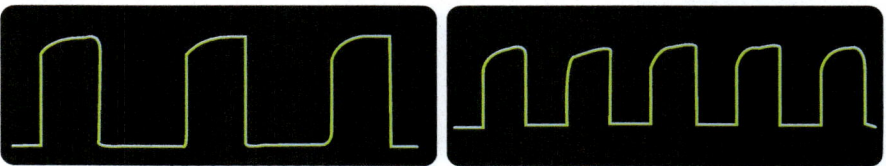

Simple pneumothorax (doesn't affect cardiac output: $P_{Et}CO_2$ rises) can be differentiated from tension pneumothorax (cardiac output falls: $P_{Et}CO_2$ falls).

It is also possible to differentiate congestive cardiac failure (CCF) from bronchospasm on the basis of the shape of the capnographic waveform: in CCF, the waveform is relatively upright.

It is possible to distinguish CHF bronchospasm on the basis of capnography.

CCF	Bronchospasm
Upright waveform	Upsloping plateau gives a 'shark fin' appearance to the waveform

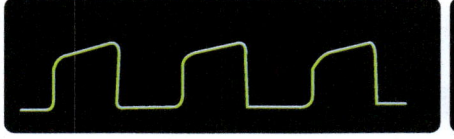 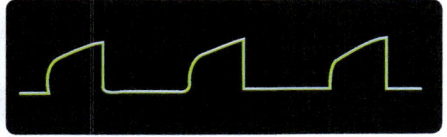

In airways obstruction (severe bronchoconstriction in an acute attack of asthma, or airway narrowing due to loss of elastic recoil in COPD), slow exhalation leads to slow CO_2-elimination results in a steeply upsloping alveolar plateau, giving a 'shark fin' appearance to the waveform. This slope correlates closely with spirometric indices of airway obstruction, making it possible to monitor bronchodilator therapy—and potentially, to estimate bronchospasm in those who cannot perform spirometry (such as patients at the extremes of age). The length of the alveolar plateau divided by the respiratory rate (the 'E_tCO_2 ratio'), closely correlates with the airway resistance.

Soto RG, Fu ES, Vila H Jr, et al. Capnography accurately detects apnea during monitored anesthesia care. Anesth Analg 2004;99(2):379–82.

Grmec S, Lah K, Tusek-Bunc K. Difference in end-tidal CO_2 between asphyxia cardiac arrest and ventricular fibrillation/pulseless ventricular tachycardia cardiac arrest in the prehospital setting. Crit Care. 2003;7:R139–44.

Kodali BS. Factors influencing $P_{Et}CO_2$. 2007. Welcome to capnography.com. Last accessed 6 June 2012.

Krauss B, Deykin A, Lam A, et al. Capnogram shape in obstructive lung disease. Anesth Analg 2005;100(3):884–8.

Kunkov S, Pinedo V, Silver EJ, et al. Predicting the need for hospitalization in acute childhood asthma using end–tidal capnography. Pediatr Emerg Care 2005;21(9):574–7.

Yaron M, Padyk P, Hutsinpiller M, et al. Utility of the expiratory capnogram in the assessment of bronchospasm. Ann Emerg Med 1996;28(4):403–7.

2.36   Esophageal Intubation

2

Unrecognized placement of the endotracheal tube (ETT) into the esophagus can prove catastrophic. None of the checks that are routinely performed to ascertain correct placement of the tube are infallible. For example, conduction of breath sounds to the chest wall is possible even though the tube may reside in the esophagus (in fact, the chest wall can still move on bagging the patient because gastric inflation can transmit some movement to the chest wall; gas exchange may even be sustained for a while because of the diaphragmatic movement so produced; a fall in the SpO_2 is often a late sign).

Conversely, the absence of breath sounds over the epigastrium does not rule out esophageal intubation.

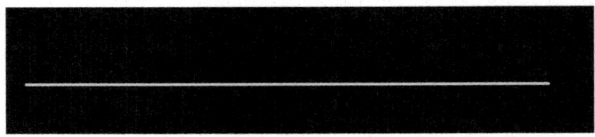

Capnograph in esophageal intubation

Carbon dioxide has its origins in the lungs. Measurable CO_2 in the ETT can only mean that the ETT resides in the tracheobronchial tree. Capnometry may be the most reliable of the available indices—short of bronchoscopic confirmation of tracheal intubation—that distinguish tracheal from esophageal intubation (Note that if the patient had initially been manually ventilated with bag and mask, some of the exhaled gas that was forced into the esophagus during bagging can be measured during the first few exhalations. On the other hand, occlusion of the tip of the ETT by cricoid pressure, applied PEEP and bronchospasm can result in failure to detect CO_2).

E_tCO_2 can help guide the ETT during a blind oral (or nasal) intubation. In a spontaneously breathing patient, a capnometer hooked to the ETT will register increase in amplitude of the EtCO$_2$ as the tube approaches the larynx, displaying the classical capnographic waveform as the ETT passes between the vocal cords.

Hasan A. Esophageal intubation. In: Understanding Mechanical Ventilation: a Practical Handbook. London: Springer; 2010. p.183, 309–10.

Ionescu T. Signs of endotracheal intubation. Anaesthesia. 1981;36:422.

Linko K, Paloheimo M and Tammisto T: Capnography for detection of accidental oesophageal intubation. Acta Anaesthesiol Scand. 1983;27:199–202.

Murry IP, Modell JH. Early detection of endotracheal tube accidents by monitoring carbon dioxide concentration in respiratory gas. Anesthesiology. 1986;59:344–6.

2.37   Capnography in Tube Disconnection and Cuff Rupture

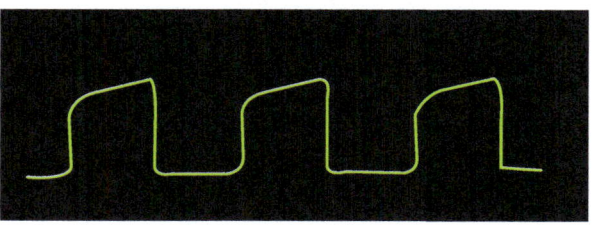

Normal capnograph

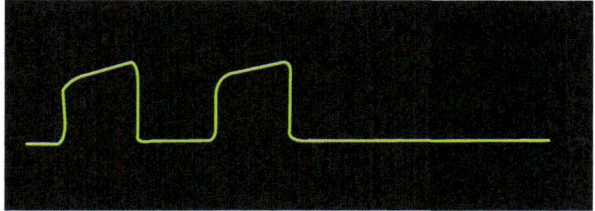

Capnograph in self-extubation or disconnection

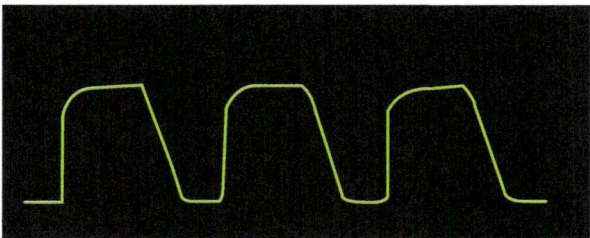

Ruptured ET cuff showing a gradual descent

2.37.1   *Biphasic Capnograph*

A biphasic pattern on the capnogram may be obtained under some circumstances, eg when there are *air leaks* in the sampling system.

In *severe kyphoscoliosis*, lung volumes and lung mechanics may considerably differ on both sides. The phases of lung emptying can therefore be out of synchrony on the two sides. Consequently, the plateau of the capnogram shows a late hump (see fig below).

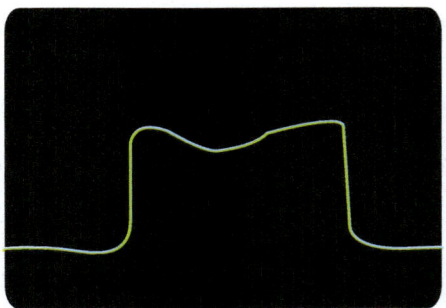

The pulsation of the heart and great vessels, by gently compressing the lungs, can produce minor changes in airflow. These *cardiac oscillations* can sometimes be recognized on the waveform, especially when the respiratory rate is low. They appear as diminutive serrations towards the end of expiration, and their frequency correlates with the heart rate (see fig below).

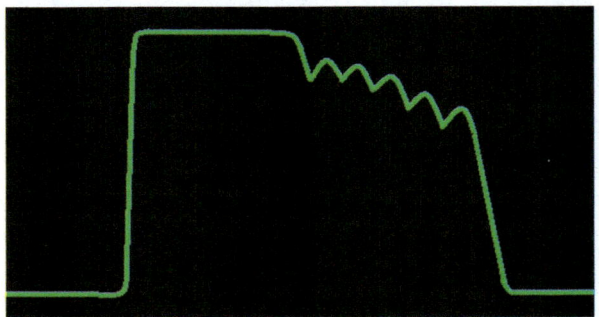

Kodali BS. Factors influencing $P_{Et}CO_2$. 2007. Welcome to capnography.com. Last accessed 6 June 2012.

References

Birmingham PK, Cheney FW, Ward RJ. Esophageal intubation: a review of detection techniques. Anesth Analg. 1986;65:886–91.

Brand TM, Brand ME, Jay GD. Enamel nail polish does not interfere with pulse oximetry. J Clin Monit Comput. 2002;17:93.

Busch MR, Mace JE, Ho NT, Ho C. Roles of the beta 146 histidine residue in the molecular basis of the Bohr effect of hemoglobin: a proton nuclear magnetic resonance study. Biochemistry. 1991;30:1865.

ECRI Health Devices Program. Carbon dioxide monitors. Health Devices. 1986;15:255–85.

Fluck Jr RR, Schroeder C, Frani G, et al. Does ambient light affect the accuracy of pulse oximetry? Respir Care. 2003;48:677.

Greene GE, Hassel KT, Mahutte CK. Comparison of arterial blood gas with continuous intraarterial and transcutaneous PO2 sensor in adult critically ill patients. Crit Care Med. 1987;15:491.

Inman KJ, Sibbald WJ, Rutledge FS. Does implementing pulse oximetry in a critical care unit result in substantial arterial blood gas savings? Chest. 1993;104:543.

Kalenda Z. Mastering infrared capnography. Utrecht, The Netherlands: Kerckebosch-Zeist, 1989:p101.

Linlo K, Paloheimo M, Tammisto T. Capnography for detection of accidental oesophageal intubation. Acta Anaesthesiol Scand. 1983;27:199–202.

Martin L, Khalil H. How much reduced hemoglobin is necessary to generate central cyanosis? Chest. 1990;97:182.

O'Flaherty D, Adams AP. The end-tidal carbon dioxide detector. Assessment of new method to distinguish oesophageal from tracheal intubation. Anaesthesia. 1990;45:653–5.

Sanders AB, Kern KB, Otto CW, et al. End-tidal carbon dioxide monitoring during cardiopulmonary resuscitation: a prognostic indicator for survival. JAMA. 1989;262:1347.

Veyckemans F, Baele P, Guillaume JE, et al. Hyperbilirubinemia does not interfere with hemoglobin saturation measured by pulse oximetry. Anesthesiology. 1989;70:118.

Zeballos RJ, Weisman IM. Reliability of noninvasive oximetry in black subjects during exercise and hypoxia. Am Rev Respir Dis. 1991;144:1240.

Chapter 3
Acids and Bases

Contents

A. Hasan, *Handbook of Blood Gas/Acid-Base Interpretation*,
DOI 10.1007/978-1-4471-4315-4_3, © Springer-Verlag London 2013

3.1   Intracellular and Extracellular pH

Most biological fluids are alkaline.

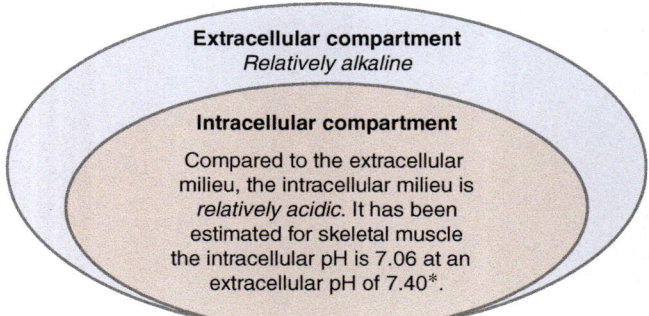

Concentrated hydrochloric acid has a pH of 1.1. The pH range found in life is 6.8–7.8. This reflects a very large range of the hydrogen ion concentration: from 16 nanomoles/L (pH 7.8) to 160 nanomoles/L (pH of 6.8).

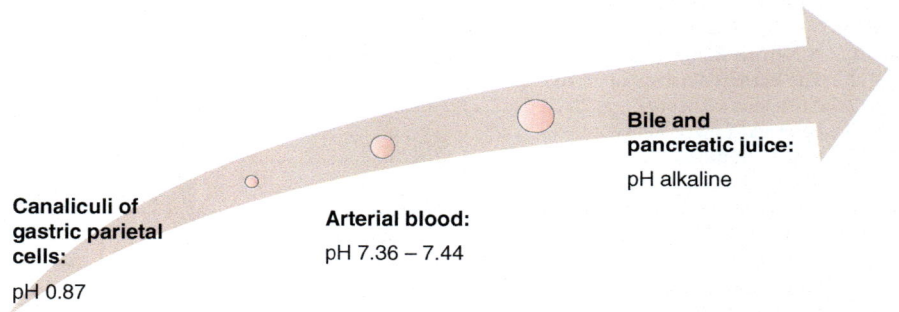

*Wray S. Smooth muscle intracellular pH: measurement, regulation, and function. Am J Physiol. 1988;254:C213.

Brandis K. Acid-base pHysiology. 2012. www.anaesthesiaMCQ.com. Last accessed 6 June 2012.

3.2   pH Differences

The intracellular microenvironment is complex, and so the pH is not uniform throughout the cell but varies between the different intracellular compartments. Since it is the cell that is the basic unit of any tissue, tissue function can best be assessed in relation to the activity of its cells.

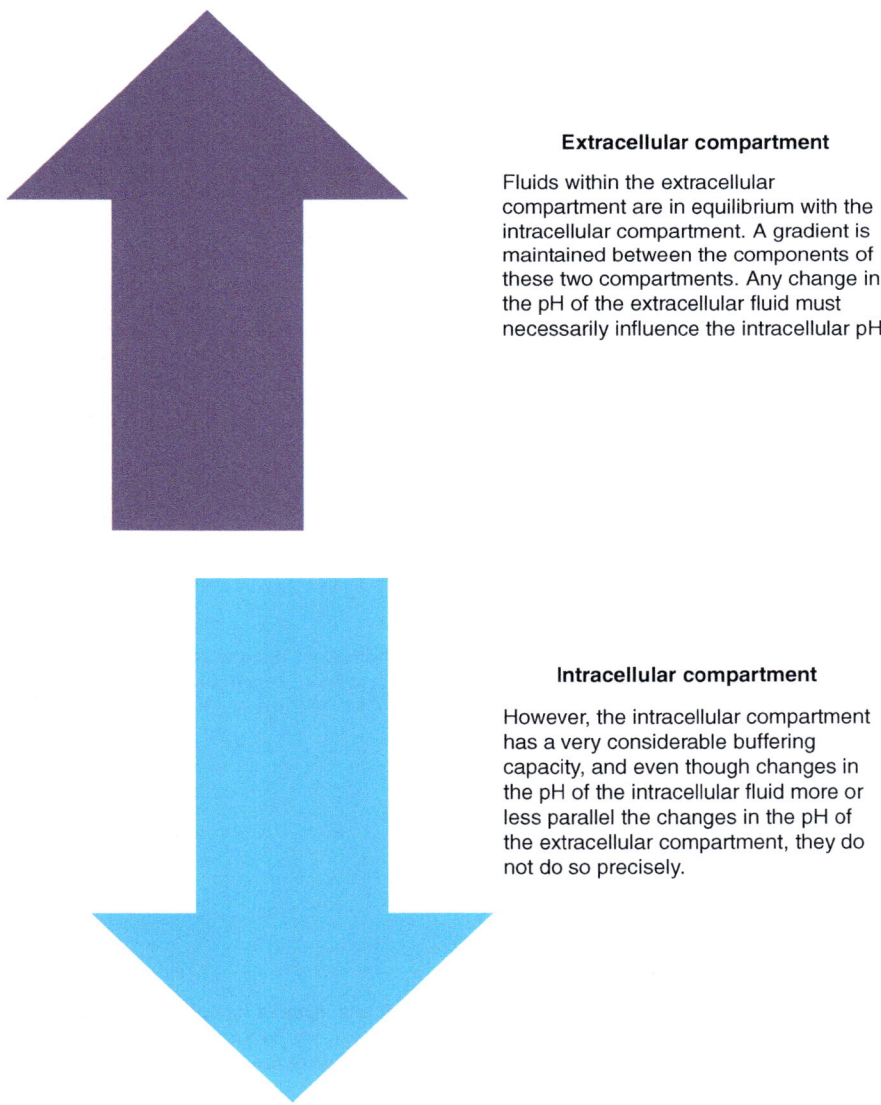

Extracellular compartment

Fluids within the extracellular compartment are in equilibrium with the intracellular compartment. A gradient is maintained between the components of these two compartments. Any change in the pH of the extracellular fluid must necessarily influence the intracellular pH.

Intracellular compartment

However, the intracellular compartment has a very considerable buffering capacity, and even though changes in the pH of the intracellular fluid more or less parallel the changes in the pH of the extracellular compartment, they do not do so precisely.

Ganapathy V, Leibach FH. Protons and regulation of biological functions. Kidney Int Suppl. 1991;33:S4.

3.3   Surrogate Measurement of Intracellular pH

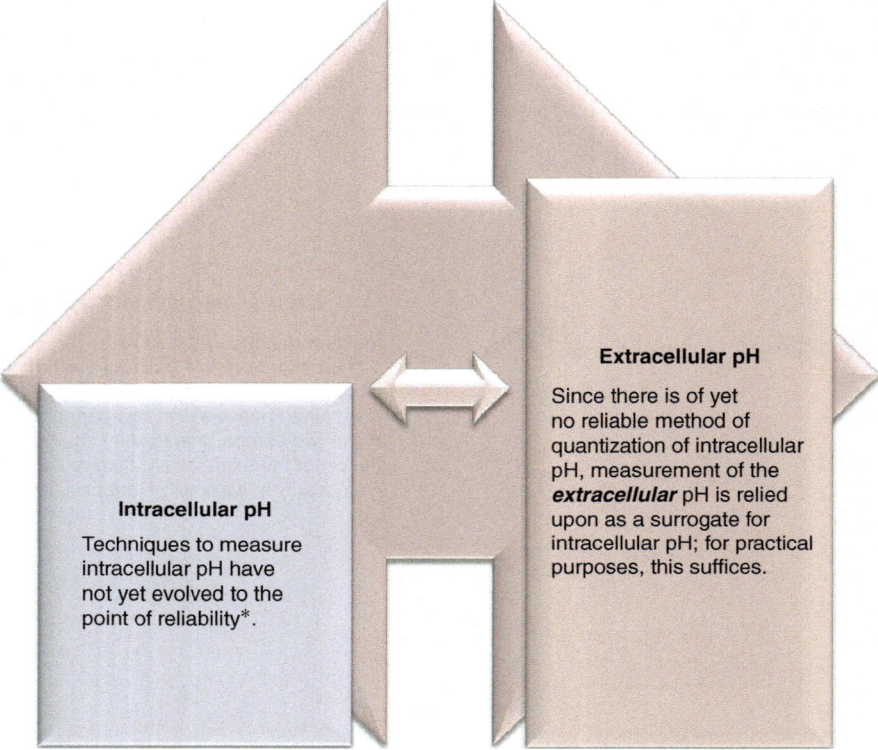

Extracellular pH

Since there is of yet
no reliable method of
quantization of intracellular
pH, measurement of the
extracellular pH is relied
upon as a surrogate for
intracellular pH; for practical
purposes, this suffices.

Intracellular pH

Techniques to measure
intracellular pH have
not yet evolved to the
point of reliability*.

*Methods such as double-tip impalement (with pH and reference microelectrodes having diameters of less than 1 μ), have been replaced with pH-dependent fluorescent dye techniques such as the 2,7-bis (carboxyethyl)-5, 6-carboxyfluorescein (BCECF) and the semi-naphthorhodafluor-1 (SNARF-1) trapped dye technique.

Carter NW, Rector FC Jr., Campion DS, Seldin DW. Measurement of intracellular pH of skeletal muscle with pH-sensitive glass microelectrodes. J Clin Invest. 1967;46(6):920–33.
Gillies RJ, Lynch RM. Frontiers in the measurement of cell and tissue pH. Novartis Found Symp. 2001;240:7–19.
Thomas RC. Intracellular pH of snail neurons measured with a new pH- sensitive glass microelectrode. J Physiol. 1974;238(1):159–80.

3.4   Preferential Permeability of the Cell Membrane

The intracellular microenvironment is protected by the cell membrane which is preferentially permeable to certain molecules only.

The *selective* permeability of the cell membrane is one of the mechanisms that help maintain a concentration gradient between the intracellular and extracellular compartments. Other mechanisms exist also.

3

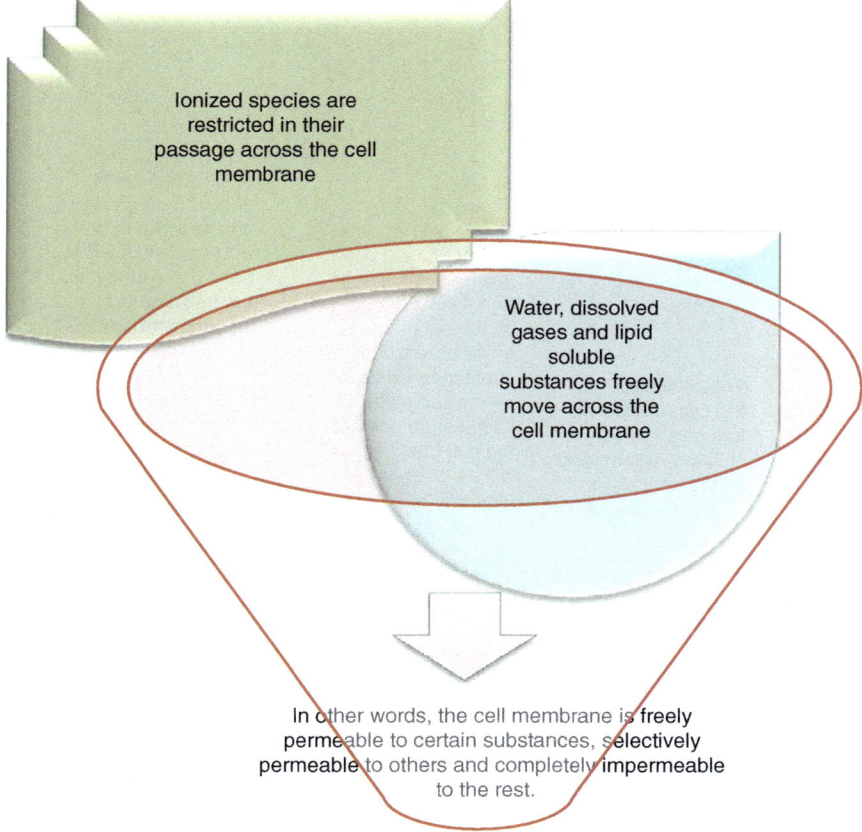

Ionized species are restricted in their passage across the cell membrane

Water, dissolved gases and lipid soluble substances freely move across the cell membrane

In other words, the cell membrane is freely permeable to certain substances, selectively permeable to others and completely impermeable to the rest.

Davis BD. On the importance of being ionized. Arch Biochem Biophys. 1958;78:497–509.

3.5   Ionization and Permeability

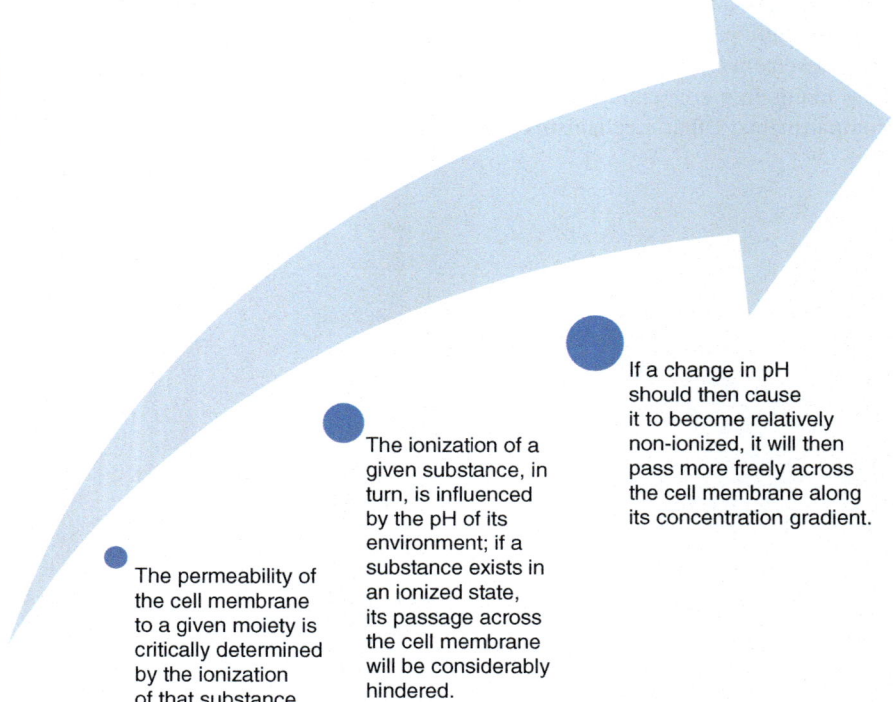

The permeability of the cell membrane to a given moiety is critically determined by the ionization of that substance.

The ionization of a given substance, in turn, is influenced by the pH of its environment; if a substance exists in an ionized state, its passage across the cell membrane will be considerably hindered.

If a change in pH should then cause it to become relatively non-ionized, it will then pass more freely across the cell membrane along its concentration gradient.

Davis BD. On the importance of being ionized. Arch Biochem Biophys. 1958;78:497–509.

3.6   The Reason Why Substances Need to Be Ionized

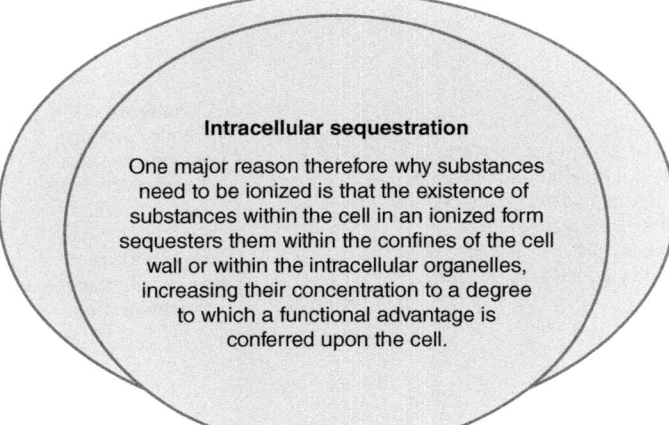

Intracellular sequestration

One major reason therefore why substances need to be ionized is that the existence of substances within the cell in an ionized form sequesters them within the confines of the cell wall or within the intracellular organelles, increasing their concentration to a degree to which a functional advantage is conferred upon the cell.

At neutral pH (7.0, which is close to the pH of most cells), barring a few exceptions, all substances exist in highly ionized states. At neutral pH (again, barring these exceptions), all *low*-molecular-weight and water-soluble substances carry ionized groups (such as phosphate, ammonium and carboxylate). Thus ionized, these low-molecular-weight and water-soluble moieties are prevented from diffusing into the extracellular fluid.

Davis BD. On the importance of being ionized. Arch Biochem Biophys. 1958;78:497–509.

3.7   The Exceptions to the Rule

Intracellular macromolecules do not need to be ionized to be retained within the cell: their very size retains them within the cell, so they do not exist in an ionic form.

Similarly lipids are mostly protein bound, and well anchored within the cell, and do not need to be highly ionized to reach high concentrations intracellularly.

On the contrary, the end products of metabolism need free egress out of the cell so that they may be excreted, and it would disadvantage the cell were they to be ionized and therefore trapped inside the cell.

Davis BD. On the importance of being ionized. Arch Biochem Biophys. 1958;78:497–509.

3.8   The Hydrogen Ion (H⁺, Proton)

The hydrogen *ion* (proton) is a hydrogen *atom* that is shorn of its sole electron. Strictly speaking, protons cannot exist as H^+ in body fluids but rather combine with water to form hydronium ions such as H_3O^+ and H_5O_2. It is for the sake of convenience that protons are represented as H^+ in chemical reactions.

3

> **The bare proton, H⁺, is very small in size (it has a radius of 1/10,000 that of the hydrogen atom).**
>
> H⁺ ions are strongly drawn to molecules such as proteins, and can therefore penetrate deeply into cellular structures and into the matrix of the protein macromolecules themselves, reaching the active sites there.
>
> Their minute size also enables tighter bonding to the negatively charged proteins, producing configurational changes within the latter. This has considerable bearing upon many vital enzymatic reactions. Cellular function can be markedly influenced by the hydrogen ion concentration of the intracellular milieu.

By ionizing intracellular protein molecules H^+ critically influences the function of:

Enzymes	Peptide hormones	Hormone receptors
Ion channels	Transporters	Mediator proteins

It is obvious therefore that the pH of the extracellular space (which is but an extension of the intracellular space) needs to be tightly regulated *in-vivo* to prevent molecular dysfunction.

Ganapathy V, Leibach FH. Protons and regulation of biological functions. Kidney Int Suppl. 1991;33:S4.

3.9   Intracellular pH Is Regulated Within a Narrow Range

Intracellular pH is determines the degree to which intracellular molecules are ionized.

Intracellular pH affects the functioning of small and large molecules.

Small molecules

Being minute, small molecules can easily be lost from the cells.

Large molecules

Macromolecules are not as susceptible to being lost out of the cell. Macromolecules are also polarized, but for a different reason.

Ionization of vital small molecules ensures their sequestration within cells, since they remain trapped by electrical gradients.

Ionization of parts of large molecules (e.g. The amino acid residues of enzymes) influences their activity.

Thus, intracellular reactions are critically dependent upon pH; this is the reason that pH needs to be regulated within narrow limits.

Ganapathy V, Leibach FH. Protons and regulation of biological functions. Kidney Int Suppl. 1991;33:S4.

3.10   A Narrow Range of pH Does Not Mean a Small Range of the H⁺ Concentration

Protein molecules are components of ion channels and their transporters, and of peptide hormones and their receptors. The function of all these substances is exquisitely sensitive to changes in pH.

3

Life is only possible between a pH range of 6. 8 – 7. 8 (or between 16 – 160 nanomoles of H⁺ per liter)

Any change in the hydrogen ion concentration has a profound impact upon biological compounds since the ionic groups that they possess (e.g., phosphate, ammonium and carboxylate) function as conjugate bases.

A pH of 6.8 corresponds to a H⁺ ion concentration of 160 nmol/L

A pH of 7.8 corresponds to a H⁺ ion concentration of 16 nmol/L

Equivalent values of pH and H⁺	
pH	$[H^+]$ (nanomoles/l)
6.8	158
6.9	125
7.0	100
7.1	79
7.2	63
7.3	50
7.4	40
7.5	31
7.6	25
7.7	20
7.8	15

As is apparent, a narrow pH range does not mean a narrow range of hydrogen ion concentration: within the apparently narrow range of 6.8–7.8 the H⁺ ion concentration can (vary) 100-fold.

Ganapathy V, Leibach FH. Protons and regulation of biological functions. Kidney Int Suppl. 1991;33:S4.

3.11   The Earliest Concept of an Acid

(Latin *acidus* = sour):

   The term acid derives from its Latin root *acidus,* meaning sour. The hallmarks of an acid were considered to be:

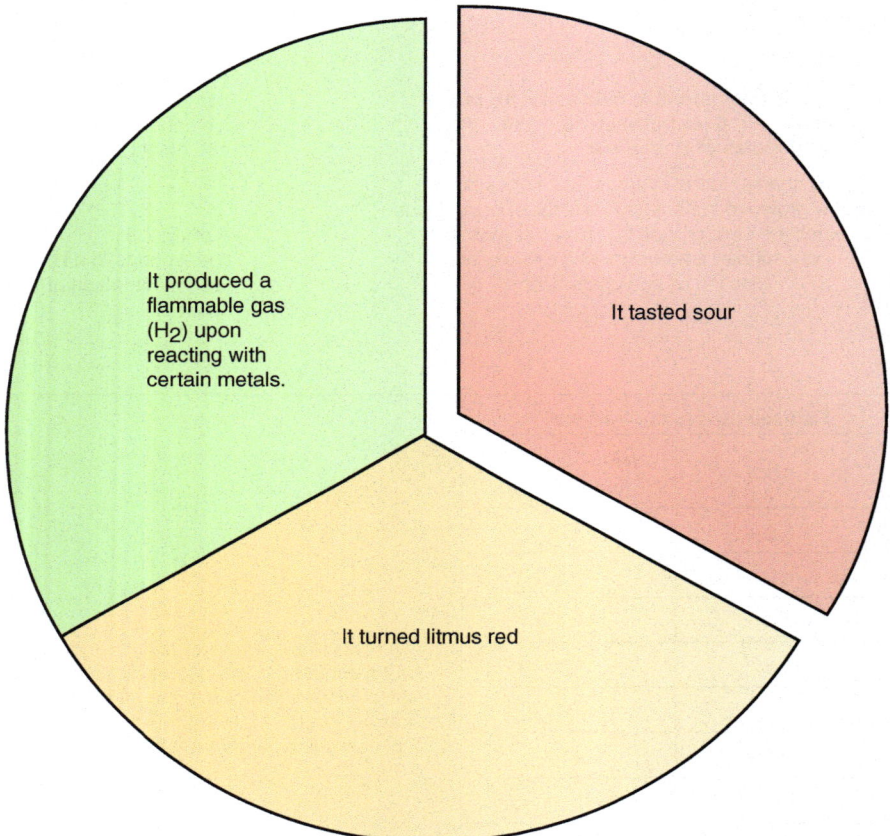

It produced a flammable gas (H_2) upon reacting with certain metals.

It tasted sour

It turned litmus red

Relman AS. What are "acids" and "bases"? Am J Med. 1954;17:435.

Rose BD, Post TW. Clinical physiology of acid-base and electrolyte disorders. 5th ed. New York: McGraw-Hill; 2001. p. 328–47.

3.12   Arrhenius's Theory

In 1887, Svante August Arrhenius redefined an acid. Although it was a vast improvement upon the existing definitions of acids and bases at that time, the theory of Arrhenius could only apply to aqueous solutions.

3

Acid: A substance that dissociates in water to produce hydrogen ions.

Base: A substance that dissociates in water to produce hydroxyl ions.

Arrhenius's acids and bases

Advantages

Arrhenius' theory was the first truly modern approach to acid-base physiology.

Disadvantages

Contrary to Arrhenius's definition of an acid, certain substances with obvious acidic properties (e.g. CO_2) do not dissociate into hydrogen ions. Again, contrary to Arrhenius's definition of a base, a few hydroxyl-lacking moieties can function as bases. Within the framework of Arrhenius' concept, acids and bases can only function in solution.

Relman AS. What are "acids" and "bases"? Am J Med. 1954;17:435.
Severinghaus JW, Astrup P. History of blood gas analysis. Int Anesthesiol Clin. 1987;25:1–224.

3.13   Bronsted-Lowry Acids

Improving upon Arrhenius' theory, Bronsted and Lowry in 1923 envisaged an acid as a proton donor and a base as a hydrogen ion acceptor, thus extending the scope of these beyond aqueous media. According to the Bronsted-Lowry concept, upon losing a proton, an acid becomes a conjugate base (so considered because it is capable of accepting a H^+ ion to form an acid).

Acid: **An H^+ ion donor**	**Conjugate base:** **An H^+ ion acceptor** **(accepts H^+ from the acid).**

Bronsted – Lowry's acids and bases

Advantages	*Disadvantages*
The B-L theory overcomes the disadvantages of the Arrhenius' definition inasmuch as, to function as an acid, an entity does not necessarily require an aqueous solution. *The BL theory is now the universally applied clinical approach.*	CO_2 has distinct acidic properties. Yet CO_2 does not fulfil the definition of a B-L acid: CO_2 contains no H^+ ions; obviously therefore, it cannot donate protons. (This difficulty can be surmounted by viewing CO_2 as part of the carbonic acid system: see later).

Brandis K. Acid-base physiology. 2012. www.anaesthesiaMCQ.com. Last accessed 6 June 2012.
Relman AS. What are "acids" and "bases"? Am J Med. 1954;17:435.

3.14   Lewis' Approach

In that same year (1923), Lewis proposed his approach in which H^+ itself was defined an acid.

3

Acid:	Base:
A potential acceptor of a pair of electrons (with the Lewis approach, H^+ itself became identified as an acid).	A potential donor of a pair of electrons.

Lewis's acids and bases	

Advantages	Disadvantages
Lewis' definition overcame the drawback of B-L theory: CO_2 could now be encompassed within the definition of an acid.	The electron concept is an uncomfortable one for clinicians!

3.15   The Usanovich Theory

In 1939 Usanovich developed his unified theory:

Usanovich's acids and bases			
Acid:		Base:	
An acid could be either of the following		A base could be either of the following	
A substance that donated a cation.	A substance that accepted an anion.	A substance that donated an anion.	A substance that accepted a cation.

Brandis K. Acid-base physiology. 2012. www.anaesthesiaMCQ.com. Last accessed 6 June 2012.
Relman AS. What are "acids" and "bases"? Am J Med. 1954;17:435.

3.16   Summary of Definitions of Acids and Bases

3

	Acid	Base
Traditional	Sour in taste Turns blue litmus red Produces a flammable gas on reacting with certain metals	Bitter in taste Turns red litmus blue Soapy to touch
Arrhenius	Dissociates to produce H^+ in aqueous solution	Dissociates to produce OH^- in aqueous solution
Bronsted-Lowry	A donor of hydrogen ions	An acceptor of hydrogen ions
Lewis	A potential acceptor of a pair of electrons	A potential donor of a pair of electrons
Usanovich	A donor of cations or an acceptor of anions	A donor of anions or an acceptor of cations

3.17   Stewart's Physico-Chemical Approach

Peter Stewart's approach is founded upon basic physicochemical laws (the Law of Electroneutrality, the Law of Conservation of Mass and the Law of Dilution). Six simultaneous equations determine the relationship of H^+ ion to other variables:

3

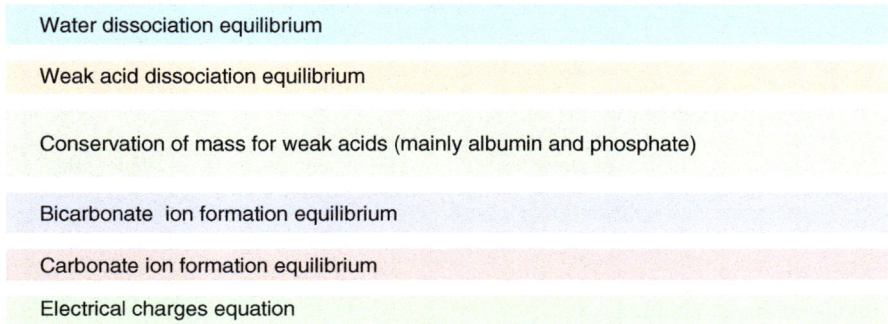

Water dissociation equilibrium

Weak acid dissociation equilibrium

Conservation of mass for weak acids (mainly albumin and phosphate)

Bicarbonate ion formation equilibrium

Carbonate ion formation equilibrium

Electrical charges equation

The fundamental principle of this approach is that, unlike in the Bronsted-Lowry approach, the bicarbonate is not an individual variable: and so the pH is not dependent upon the serum bicarbonate concentration.

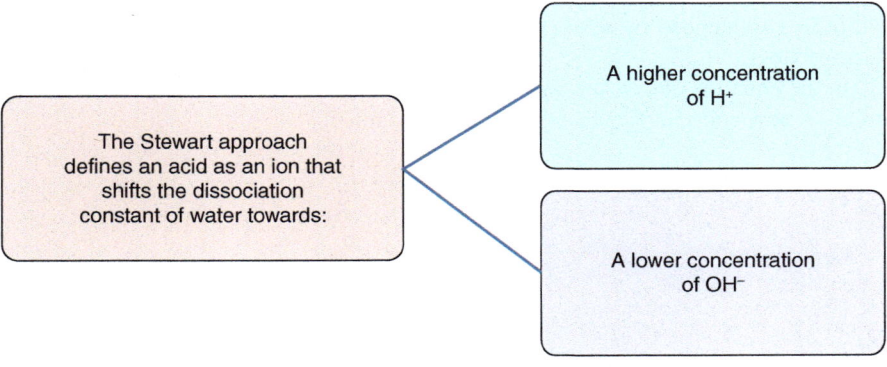

The Stewart approach defines an acid as an ion that shifts the dissociation constant of water towards:

A higher concentration of H^+

A lower concentration of OH^-

Gilfix BM, Bique M, Magder S. A physical chemical approach to the analysis of acid-base balance in the clinical setting. J Crit Care. 1993;8:187–97.

Stewart PA. How to understand acid-base. In A quantitative acid-base primer for biology and medicine. Edited by Stewart PA. Elsevier, New York, 1981:1–286.

Stewart PA. Modern quantitative acid-base chemistry. Can J Physiol Pharmacol. 1983;61:1444.

3.18   The Dissociation of Water

The unequal charge distribution on the water molecule gives it its particular physicochemical characteristics. Water is ionized into the negatively charged OH^- (hydroxyl) and the positively charged H^+ (hydrogen ion, or proton). H^+ is properly written as H_nO, given that it can exist as H_3O^+, $H_5O_2^+$ or $H_9O_4^+$ etc.

Water dissociation is the source of all H^+ and OH^- ions.

At 25 °C the ionic concentration of $[H^+]$ and $[OH^-]$ is 1.0 x 10^{-7} mEq/L. In other words, under these conditions the pH of water is 7.0.

A rise in temperature makes water acidic (pH is 6.1 at 100 °C).	A fall in temperature makes water alkaline (pH is 7.5 at 0 °C).

The pH of the blood (7.4) reflects the pH of the extracellular space. Intracellular fluid is acidic, around pH 6.9.

The dissociation of water can be represented by the following equation:

$$[H^+] \times [OH^-] = K_w \times [H_2O]$$

where, K_w is the dissociation constant of water. The numeric value of K_w is relatively small (about 4.3×10^{-16} Eq/l at 37 °C). The dissociation of water (and therefore its pH) is influenced by temperature (see above) and dissolved constituents (e.g. electrolytes).

In the equation above, the value of $[H_2O]$ is relative to the other entities is enormous; a new constant K'_w can therefore be assumed:

$$K'_w = K_w \times [H_2O]$$

Or,

$$K'_w = [H^+][OH^-]$$

In other words, if $[H^+]$ should increase, $[OH^-]$ will decrease by a similar extent.

Stewart's acids can be conceptualized as ions that drive the dissociation equilibrium of water towards a higher concentration of H^+ and a lower concentration of OH^-.

Chaplin MF. A proposal for restructuring Water. Biophys Chem. 2000;83:211–21.

Marx D, Tuckerman ME, HutterJ, Parillo M. The nature of the hydrared excess proton in water. Nature. 1999;397:601–4.

3.19   Electrolytes, Non-electrolytes and Ions

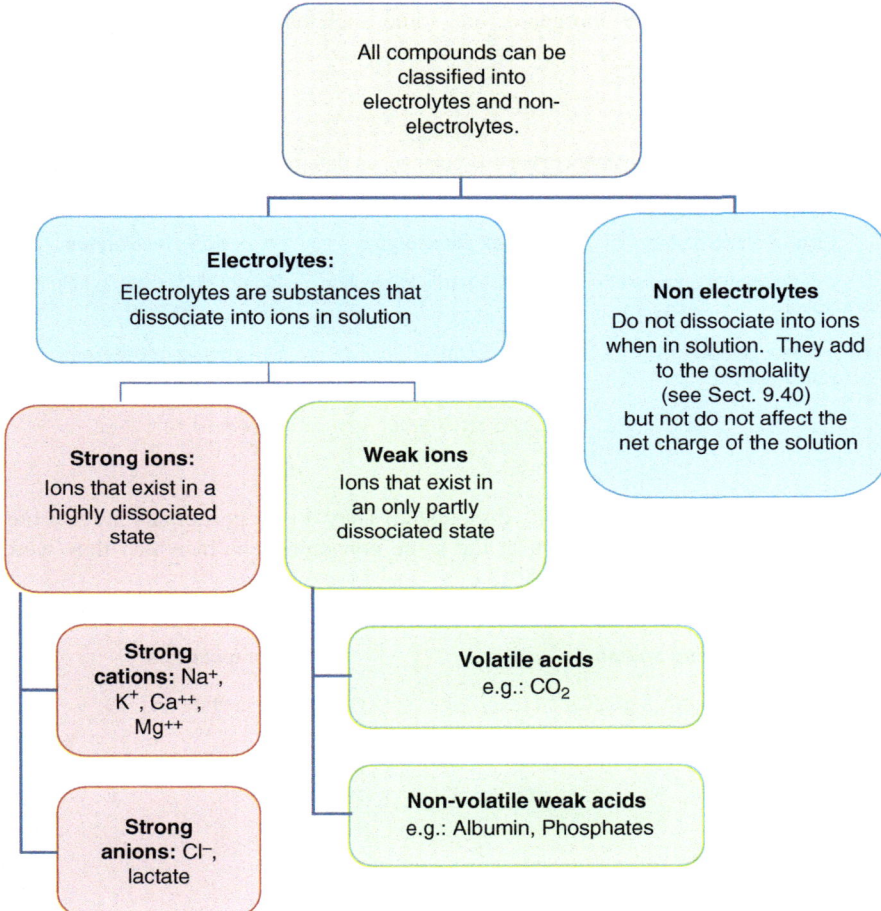

Stewart PA. How to understand acid-base. In a quantitative acid-base primer for biology and medicine. Edited by Stewart PA. Elsevier, New York, 1981:1–286.
Stewart PA. Modern quantitative acid-base chemistry. Can J Physiol Pharmacol. 1983;61:1444.

3.20   Strong Ions

Most strong anions are inorganic, but some such as lactate and sulphate are organic.

Ionization
The dissociation constants of various substances determine the degree of their ionization in solution.

Strong electrolytes	Weak electrolytes	Non electrolytes
Dissociate almost completely in solution.	Dissociate partly in solution.	Do not dissociate in solution.
Their dissociation constants are usually in excess of 10^{-4} Eq/L.	Their dissociation constants normally range between 10^{-4} Eq/L and 10^{-12} Eq/L.	Substances are defined as non-electrolytes when their dissociation constants lie below 10^{-12} Eq/L.

Strong ions are effectively fully dissociated. They do not participate in reactions and are therefore always present at the same concentrations in which they were added to the system.

Strong anions	Strong cations
Na^+; also: K^+, Mg^{++}, Ca^{++}	Cl^- (less so: lactate and SO_4^-)

Brandis K. Acid-base pHysiology; www.anaesthesiaMCQ.com. Last accessed 6 June 2012.

Stewart PA. How to understand acid-base. In a quantitative acid-base primer for biology and medicine. Edited by Stewart PA. Elsevier, New York, 1981:1–286.

Stewart PA. Modern quantitative acid-base chemistry. Can J Physiol Pharmacol. 1983;61:1444.

3.21 Stewart's Determinants of the Acid Base Status

Peter Stewart described *Independent Variables* as "…those which can be directly altered from outside the system without affecting each other", and *Dependent Variables* as those "…internal to the system. Their values represent the system's reaction to the externally imposed values of the independent variables."

Three independent variables determine the acid base status:

PaCO$_2$	The strong-ion difference (SID)	A$_{tot}$
The partial pressure of CO$_2$ in the plasma (solution).	The difference between the sum of the strong anions and strong cations.	The concentration of non volatile weak acids/buffers in the solution (plasma): Mainly *albumin* (or rather, the ionic equivalence of the plasma albumin concentration) and *phosphates*.

Based on this, six primary acid-base disturbances are possible:

Respiratory acidosis	Respiratory alkalosis	Strong ion acidosis	Strong ion alkalosis	Non-volatile buffer acidosis	Non-volatile buffer alkalosis

Note that pH is a *dependent* variable.

Corey HE. Bench-to-bedside review: Fundamental principles of acid-base physiology. Crit Care. 2005;9:184–92.

Gilfix BM, Bique M, Magder S. A physical chemical approach to the analysis of acid-base balance in the clinical setting. J Crit Care. 1993;8:187–97.

Stewart PA. How to understand acid-base. In a quantitative acid-base primer for biology and medicine. Edited by Stewart PA. Elsevier, New York, 1981:1–286.

Stewart PA. Modern quantitative acid-base chemistry. Can J Physiol Pharmacol. 1983;61:1444.

3.22 Apparent and Effective Strong Ion Difference

Strong Ion Difference (SID)

SID is the difference between the sum of the strong (completely dissociated) cations and the sum of the strong (completely dissociated) anions.

$$SID = strong\ cations - strong\ anions$$

(In practice, SID is never precisely quantified because all strong ions are not measurable.)

Apparent Strong Ion Difference (SID$_{app}$)

SID$_{app}$ is the difference between the **sum of the measurable strong cations** and the **sum of the measurable strong anions.**

SID$_{app}$ = ([Na] + [K] + [ionized Ca] + [ionized Mg]) − ([Cl] + [Lactate]).

SID$_{app}$ is normally 40 mEq/L. SID$_{app}$ greater than this is considered indicative of metabolic acidosis.

Effective Strong Ion Difference (SID$_{eff}$)

Based on the *Law of Electroneutrality* (09.03), the difference between the cations and anions should be balanced by the weak acids and CO_2; the latter two therefore, may equally be used to calculate the SID*

Thus, *SID$_{eff}$ is a function of:*

pH

A$_{tot}$

The two major determinants of A$_{tot}$ are:

- *Albumin:* the ion equivalence of albumin concentration.
- *Phosphates* (comprise less than 5 % of A$_{tot}$ and can usually be ignored).

*Conceptually, this makes the SID$_{eff}$ the equivalent of the known buffer base.

Corey HE. Bench-to-bedside review: Fundamental principles of acid-base physiology. Crit Care. 2005;9:184–92.

Gilfix BM, Bique M, Magder S. A physical chemical approach to the analysis of acid-base balance in the clinical setting. J Crit Care. 1993;8:187–97.

3.23   Strong Ion Gap

$$SID = [Na^+ + K^+] - [Cl^- + lactate]$$

Because all strong ions are not measurable, the SID is not directly calculable.

The apparent SID (SID$_{app}$)	**The effective SID (SID$_{eff}$)**
Calculated using concentrations available **strong cations (Na$^+$, K$^+$, ionized Ca, ionized Mg)**, and **strong anions (Cl$^-$, lactate)** in blood.	Calculated using CO_2, albumin, and phosphate

The **Strong Ion Gap (SIG)** is the difference between these two ways of measuring the SID:

$$SIG = SID_{app} - SID_{eff}$$

It is thus a quantification of unmeasured anions (both strong and weak) and thus, identical to the Buffer Base of Singer and Hastings (9.23).

Normally, (in the absence of unmeasured ions),

$$SID_{eff} = SID_{app} = SID_{eff}$$

and so the difference between the two (namely the strong ion gap) should be zero (Normal SIG: 0 mEq/L). In practice, this situation is exceptional.

If the value of SID is changed, more or less water will dissociate (to maintain electroneutrality): the hydrogen ion concentration will resultantly change. *An increase in the strong ion difference* will increase blood pH, whereas *a decrease in the strong ion difference* will decrease it.

Compared to the anion gap (AG), the SIG is possibly a superior measure of unmeasured anions. For instance, the SIG will be high in hypoalbuminemia revealing a disorder that can potentially widen the AG, at a time when the *uncorrected* AG itself is normal.

Based on these independent variables, acid-base disorders can be classified (see Sect. 3.24).

Chatburn RL, Mireles-Cabodevila E. Handbook of respiratory care. Sudbury, Mass.: Jones & Bartlett Learning (3rd edition); 2011. p. 81–3.

Corey HE. Bench-to-bedside review: Fundamental principles of acid-base physiology. Crit Care. 2005;9:184–92.

3.24   Major Regulators of Independent Variables

Respiratory variables	Metabolic variables		
PaCO$_2$	**SID**		**A$_{tot}$**
The H$^+$ concentration changes consequent to changes in PaCO$_2$.	**Change in dilution**	**Changes in strong ion concentration**	Changes in concentration of phosphate, albumin, and other plasma proteins. In vivo, weak acids ("buffers") exist either in a dissociated state (A$^-$), or in association with a proton (AH). $A_{tot} = [A^-] + [AH]$ The major contributor to the ionic charge of weak acids is albumin (and to a much smaller extent, phosphate).
	Dehydration: -SID increases -Alkalinity increases	*Accumulation of inorganic acids:* -Cl$^-$ increases -SID low, SIG low	
	Water overload: -SID decreases -Alkalinity decreases.	*Accumulation of organic acids (lactate, formate, or ketones):* -SID low, SIG high.	
The major external regulator is the lung. Changes in ventilation can produce large changes in CO$_2$ rapidly. CO$_2$ is rapidly diffusible across all biological membranes.	The major external regulator is the kidney through its excretion of ions. The gut also influences the concentration of ions by regulating their absorption. Renal secretory processes are relatively slow. Strong ions however can cross biological membranes with relative ease.		The major external regulator of albumin is the liver. The production of albumin by the liver is relatively slow. Also albumin being a large molecule cannot transit biological membrane rapidly.
Rapid	**Relatively slow**		**Slowest**

Chatburn RL, Mireles-Cabodevila E. Handbook of respiratory care. Sudbury, Mass.: Jones & Bartlett Learning (3rd edition); 2011. p. 81–3.

Corey HE. Bench-to-bedside review: fundamental principles of acid-base physiology. Crit Care. 2005;9:184–92.

3.25   Fourth Order Polynomial Equation

From the set of the six simultaneous equations, a fourth order polynomial equation is derived. Though complex and often befuddling to clinicians, the equation can be quickly solved on computers.

3

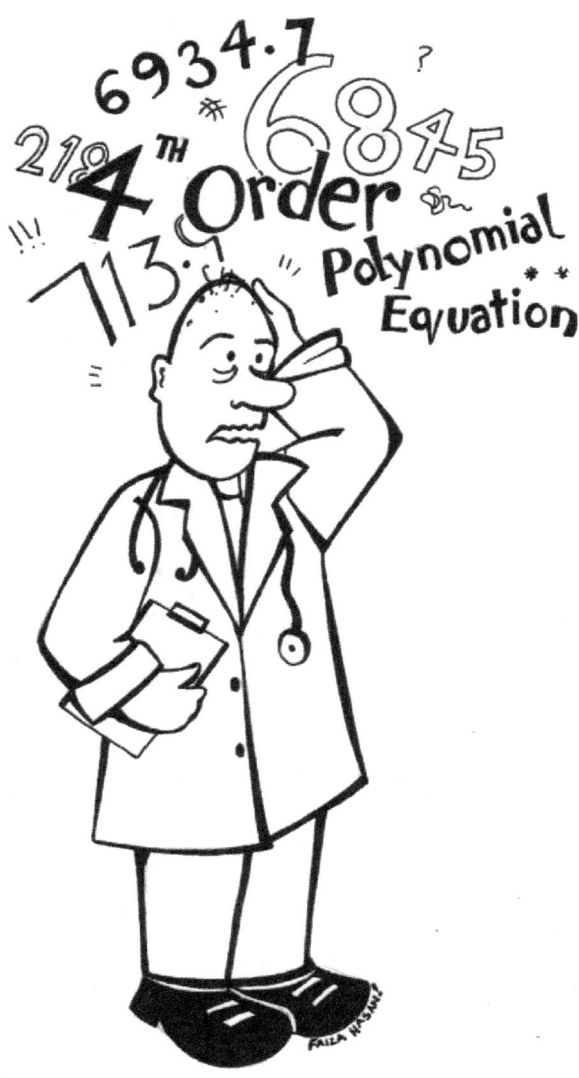

Water dissociation equilibrium	$[H^+] \times [OH^-] = K'w$
Weak acid dissociation equilibrium	$[H^+] \times [A^-] = Ka \times [HA]$
Conservation of mass for A^-	$[A_{tot}] = [HA] + [A^-]$
Bicarbonate ion formation equilibrium	$[H^+] \times [HCO_3^-] = K'1 \times S \times PaCO_2$
Carbonate ion formation equilibrium	$[H^+] \times [CO_3^-] = K3 \times [HCO_3^-]$
Electrical charges equation	$[SID^+] = [HCO_3^-] + [A^-] + [CO_3^-] + [OH^-] - [H^+]$

3.26   The Workings of Stewart's Approach

Stewart's acids are ions that shift the dissociation equilibrium of water towards a higher concentration of H^+ and a lower concentration of OH^-.

As per Stewart's approach, neither the bicarbonate nor the hydrogen ion concentrations play a direct role in determining pH, and this can be illustrated by the following examples which have to do with the concentration of chloride (a strong anion).

3

Loss of Chloride ions	Gain of Chloride ions
Example: Vomiting or continuous nasogastric aspiration	*Example:* Sodium chloride infusion
The loss of chloride (a strong anion), increases the SID_{app}, resulting in alkalosis	(NaCl solution contains equal proportions of strong cations (Na^+) as well as a strong anion(Cl^-), and has a SID of zero). Addition of a zero-SID solution will reduce thevalue of the SID_{app} of blood to below 40 mEq/L (40 mEq/L is the normal SID_{app} of blood), consequently acidifying the blood.
As per the Stewart approach, it is the loss of Cl^- and not the loss of H^+ that is responsible for gastric aspiration-related alkalosis.	As per the Stewart approach, it is the gain of Cl^- rather than dilution of the bicarbonate that is responsible for the saline infusion-related acidosis.

The Stewart approaches takes into consideration the serum albumin concentration, which the traditional approach does not (unless the corrected anion gap is used – see Sect. 9.9) and herein lies the difference between the two. Because of the intricacies of the calculations involved in the Stewart approach, computer-based calculators have been developed, which rapidly compute the results upon entering the various components of the six equations.

Chapter 4
Buffer Systems

4

Contents

A. Hasan, *Handbook of Blood Gas/Acid-Base Interpretation*,
DOI 10.1007/978-1-4471-4315-4_4, © Springer-Verlag London 2013

4.1   Generation of Acids

As a consequence of metabolic reactions in the body, considerable quantities of acid (and somewhat smaller quantities of base) are constantly being produced. Acids are generated from the metabolism of sulphur containing amino acids (e.g. methionine and cystine) and cationic amino acids (arginine and lysine).

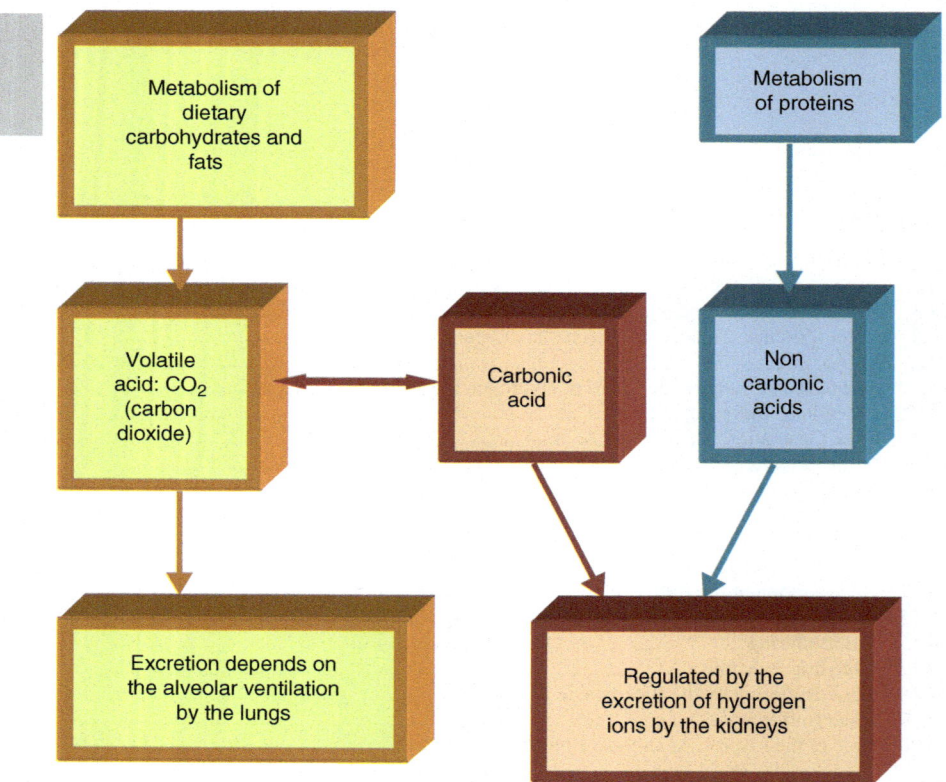

Halperin ML, Jungas RL. The metabolic production and renal disposal of hydrogen ions: an examination of the biochemical processes. Kidney Int. 1983;24:709.

Kurtz I, Maher T, Hulter HN. Effect of diet on plasma acid-base composition in normal humans. Kidney Int. 1983;24:670.

4.2   Disposal of Volatile Acids

Basal CO_2 production

Under basal conditions, about 12,000 mmol of CO_2 are produced per day.

CO_2 production: about 200 ml per minute

i.e $200 \times 60 \times 24$ ml = 288 litres per day

Since each gram-molecule of CO_2 takes up a volume of 22.4 litres at STP,

CO_2 production = 12 moles/day

With usual levels of activity CO_2 production ranges between 15,000–20,000 mmol/day.

Changes in alveolar ventilation can rapidly alter intracellular pH.

Being highly lipid-soluble, CO_2 can easily diffuse across biological membranes.

Large changes in alveolar ventilation can dramatically alter intracellular pH.

CO_2 fluctuations can have an instantaneous and powerful effect on intracellular pH (and therefore on cellular metabolism) of all body tissues.

4

Grogono AW. Acid-Base Tutorial http://www.acid-base.com/production.php. Last accessed 6 June 2012.

4.3   Disposal of Fixed Acids

Although lungs quantitatively excrete more acid, there is no way to excrete fixed acids except through the kidney.

$$H_2CO_3 \rightleftharpoons [H^+] + [HCO_3^-]$$

The urinary loss of a single filtered HCO_3^- ion is equivalent to the gain of a proton.

Therefore all the filtered HCO_3^- (which is about 4,300* mEq!) needs to be absorbed before the excretion of the daily dietary load of H^+ (50–100 mEq).

90 % of the filtered bicarbonate is reabsorbed in the proximal convoluted tubule; the rest is absorbed by the distal convoluted tubules and the collecting ducts.

50–100 mEq (average 70 mEq) of fixed acids are excreted daily through the urine. In states of increased acid production the kidney is capable of gradually stepping up the $[H^+]$ excretion to over 300 mEq per day. This is mainly acheived by NH_4 excretion. The renal response is slow and takes about 4 days to reach its maximum.

H^+ excretion in the urine is capable of a tenfold rise.	A urinary pH of as low as 4.5 can be achieved.	The H^+ gradient across the tubular membranes can increase up to a thousandfold.

*Daily filtered bicarbonate $=$ GFR $\times$ plasma bicarbonate concentration

$= 180$ L/day $\times 24$ mmol/L

$= 4,320$ mmol/day (i.e., 4,000–5,000 mmol per day).

Grogono AW. Acid-Base Tutorial http://www.acid-base.com/production.php. Last accessed 6 June 2012.

Halperin ML, Jungas RL. The metabolic production and renal disposal of hydrogen ions: an examination of the biochemical processes. Kidney Int. 1983;24:709.

Malnic G, Giebisch G. Mechanism of renal hydrogen ion secretion. Kidney Int. 1972;1:280.

4.4   Buffer Systems

Biologic fluids have in-built systems to defend their pH against changes produced by chemical reactions. Since most enzymes operate effectively only within narrow ranges of the hydrogen ion concentration, changes in pH may adversely affect their functioning.

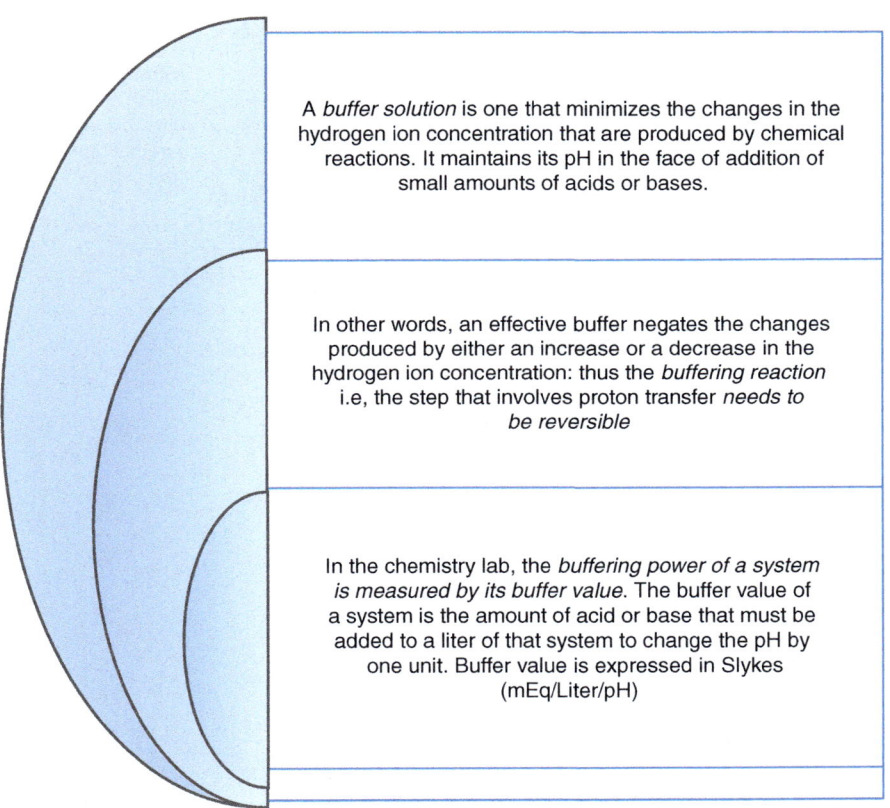

A *buffer solution* is one that minimizes the changes in the hydrogen ion concentration that are produced by chemical reactions. It maintains its pH in the face of addition of small amounts of acids or bases.

In other words, an effective buffer negates the changes produced by either an increase or a decrease in the hydrogen ion concentration: thus the *buffering reaction* i.e, the step that involves proton transfer *needs to be reversible*

In the chemistry lab, the *buffering power of a system is measured by its buffer value*. The buffer value of a system is the amount of acid or base that must be added to a liter of that system to change the pH by one unit. Buffer value is expressed in Slykes (mEq/Liter/pH)

4

4.5 Buffers

Enzymatic reactions function within a narrow range of pH: buffers are very important for *immediate* neutralization of body acid. Buffers can be:

Mixtures of weak acids with their alkali salts:

In the body buffer systems are of this nature. Salts of strong acids (such as Sodium Chloride) make poor buffers; at the usual body pH, they exhibit a high degree of ionization, and therefore have a poor affinity for the hydrogen ion.

Mixtures of weak bases with their acidic salts:

Strong alkalis (such as Sodium Hydroxide) are not found in the body.

Extracellular buffers

The carbonic acid-bicarbonate buffer system constitutes the most important buffer of the extracellular fluid. Carbonic acid exists in equilibrium with its alkali salts – either sodium or potassium bicarbonate.

Intracellular buffers

Important intracellular buffer comprise the phosphate buffer system and the protein buffer system (proteins with their alkali salts). The concentration of phosphates within the cell is nearly a dozen times their concentration within extracellular fluid. Consequently whereas phosphates do not play an important part in extracellular buffering, they are very effective as intracellular buffers.

Fernandez PC, Cohen RM, Feldman GM. The concept of bicarbonate distribution space: The crucial role of body buffers. Kidney Int. 1989;36:747.

4.6   Mechanisms for the Homeostasis of Hydrogen Ions

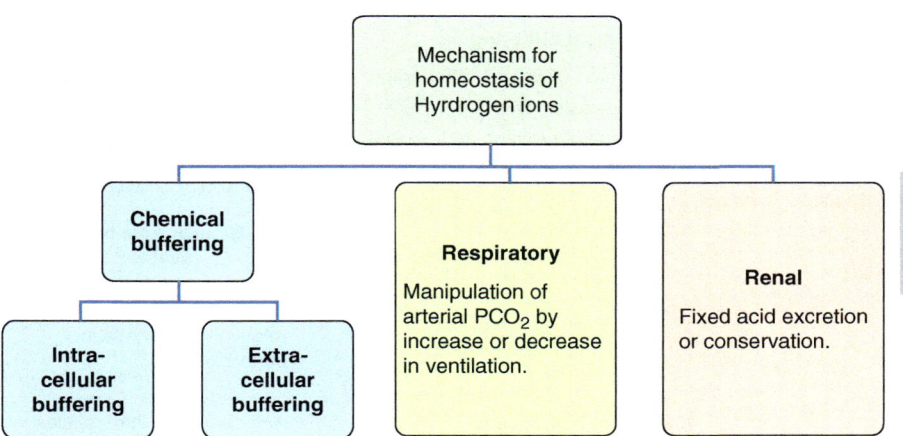

4

Fernandez PC, Cohen RM, Feldman GM. The concept of bicarbonate distribution space: the crucial role of body buffers. Kidney Int. 1989;36:747.

Hamm LL, Simon EE. Roles and mechanisms of urinary buffer excretion. Am J Physiol. 1987; 253:F595.

4.7   Intracellular Buffering

Physico-chemical buffering	**Proteins***
Of the three processes, physico-chemical buffering provides buffering of the greatest magnitude. This is because of a high intracellular concentration of proteins and phosphates, and a pK (see Sect. 5.6) which very closely approximates the intracellular pH.	E.g., the imidazole groups of histidine
	Phosphates*
	Intracellular phosphates
	Bicarbonate buffer system*
	*Intra*cellularly, this important *extra*cellular buffer plays a relatively minor role in buffering.
Metabolic buffering	Any change in intracellular pH alters intracellular enzyme pathways. This helps restore the pH towards normal.
Metabolic buffering processes are only about half as efficient as physico-chemical buffering processes.	
Organellar buffering	
H^+ can either be sequestered within or released from intracellular organelles.	

*Together, these three processes are responsible for virtually all the buffering that occurs in response to an acute acid load

Madias NE, Cohen JJ. Acid-base chemistry and buffering. In: Cohen JJ, Kassirer JP, editors. Acid-base. Boston: Little Brown; 1982.

4.8   Alkali Generation

Madias NE, Cohen JJ. Acid-base chemistry and buffering. In: Cohen JJ, Kassirer JP, editors. Acid-base. Boston: Little Brown; 1982.

4.9 Buffer Systems of the Body

Different buffer systems assume dominant roles in different parts of the body.

Extracellular fluid	*Major buffer*
	  • Bicarbonate buffer system
	Minor buffers
	  • Intracellular proteins
	  • Phosphate buffer system

Blood	*Major buffers*
	  • Bicarbonate buffer system
	  • Hemoglobin
	Minor buffers
	  • Plasma proteins
	  • Phosphate buffer system

Intracellular fluid	*Major buffers*
	  • Proteins
	  • Phosphate

Urine	*Major buffers*
	  • Ammonia
	  • Phosphate

Brandis K. Acid-base pHysiology. www.anaesthesiaMCQ.com. Last accessed 6 June 2012.

Madias NE, Cohen JJ. Acid-base chemistry and buffering. In: Cohen JJ, Kassirer JP, editors. Acid-base. Boston: Little Brown; 1982.

4.10   Transcellular Ion Shifts with Acute Acid Loading

The maintenance of pH in the face of acid loading is on account of ion fluxes across the cell membrane. The coupled exchange of ions (H^+ for HCO_3^- and Na^+ for Cl^-) is an electroneutral process; this means that the membrane potential remains unaltered.

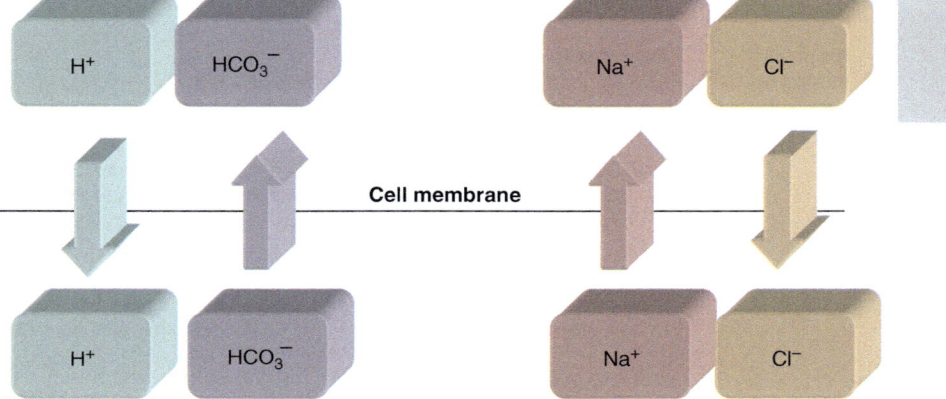

4.11   Time-Frame of Compensatory Responses to Acute Acid Loading

Immediate response	**Extracellular buffering** Principally by the bicarbonate buffer system (the non-bicarbonate buffer systems play a greater role in buffering the acidosis resulting from bicarbonate depletion).
A few minutes to several hours	**Respiratory compensation:** CO_2 washed out by increase in alveolar ventilation.
About 2–4 h	**Intracellular buffering eg:** • **RBC buffering:** The positively charged hydrogen ions enter RBC. They are accompanied by the negatively charged chloride ions. This helps maintain electroneutrality • **Bone cells:** H^+ ions enter bone cells. Na^+, K^+, and later Ca^{++} exit the bone to maintain electroneutrality. The gain of Na^+ to the ECF is relatively minor given the vast extracellular Na^+ stores. However, hyperkalemia can result owing to the K^+ migration out of bone cells.
Hours to days	**Renal compensation:** By increased tubular secretion (see Sect. 9.17).

Brandis K. Acid-base pHysiology. www.anaesthesiaMCQ.com. Last accessed 6 June 2012.

4.12   Quantifying Buffering

Buffering in metabolic acidosis

Buffering *cannot* be estimated by changes in the H+		Buffering *can* be estimated by a decrease in serum bicarbonate	
The increase in H+ is relatively small	**A⁻ is consumed in the buffering process**	Whatever the cause of the metabolic acidosis, the serum bicarbonate falls.	
The amount of acid added cannot be quantified by the increase in H+ concentration.	The decrease in A⁻ can be used to indirectly quantitate the H+ added.	**Metabolic acidosis due to acid loading**	**Metabolic acidosis due to bicarbonate loss.**
The apparent increase in H+ is only to the order of a few nanomoles.	A reduction in A⁻ by 1 mmol represents the addition of 1 million nanomol/L of H+ to the buffer system!	H+ ions react with bicarbonate and use it up.	
		Fall in serum bicarbonate	Fall in serum bicarbonate.

4

Brandis K. Acid-base pHysiology. www.anaesthesiaMCQ.com. Last accessed 6 June 2012.

Schwartz WB, Orming KJ, Porter R. The internal distribution of hydrogen ions with varying degrees of metabolic acidosis. J Clin Invest. 1957;36:373.

4.13   Buffering in Respiratory Acidosis

Compared to that in metabolic acidosis, the buffering mechanism in response to respiratory acidosis is quite different.

Extracellular buffering is ineffective in respiratory acidosis.	$$CO_2 \rightleftharpoons H_2O \rightleftharpoons H_2CO_3$$ The dominant extracellular buffer, the bicarbonate buffer system cannot buffer H_2CO_3 which is one of its own components.
Renal response is slow.	Renal compensation is relatively slow and takes several days to get established. Although slow, this is an important mechanism as once fully developed it considerably enhances the body's buffering capacity*.
Since renal compensation is relatively slow and the bicarbonate buffer system (the dominant buffer system of the extracellular space) cannot buffer H_2CO_3, **intracellular buffering becomes vital.**	**RBC** CO_2 diffuses into RBC. In a reaction catalysed by the enzyme carbonic anhydrase, it combines with water forming carbonic acid: $$CO_2 + H_2O \rightleftharpoons H_2CO_3$$ The carbonic acid reacts with haemoglobin: $$H_2CO_3 + Hb \rightleftharpoons [Hb^+] + [HCO_3^-]$$ The bicarbonate moves back into the ECF. **Bone** H^+ ions entering the bone cells are exchanged for Na^+ and K^+ ions. The Na^+ and K^+ ions move back into the ECF.

*Acutely the plasma HCO_3^- increases by 1 mmol/L for every 10 mmHg rise in PCO_2; later, once the renal response is established, it increases by about 3.5 mmol/L for a 10 mmHg increase in PCO_2.

Pitts RF. Physiology of the kidney and body fluids. Chicago: Year Book; 1974. Chapter 11.

Rose B, Post T. Buffers-II, In: www.utd.com. Last updated: Oct 6, 2010. Last accessed: 13 May 2012.

4.14 Regeneration of the Buffer

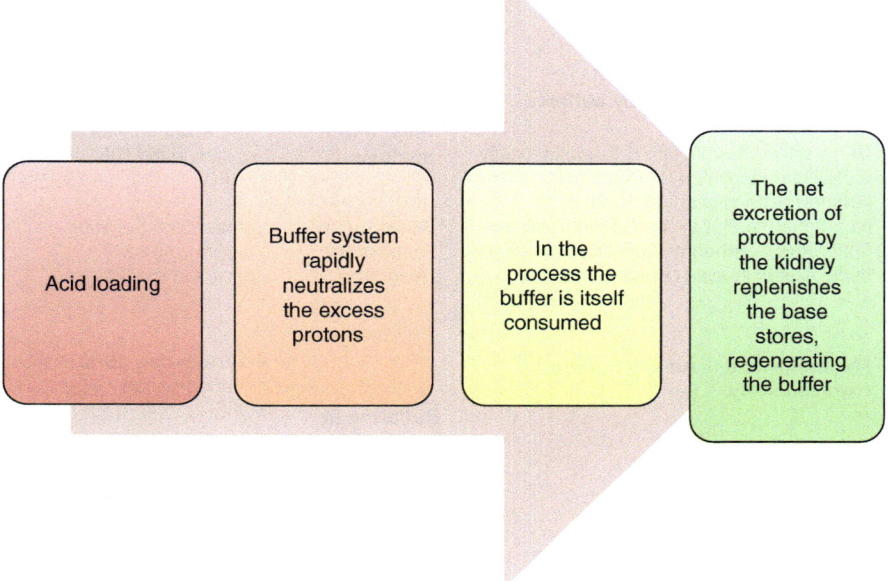

4.15 Buffering in Alkalosis

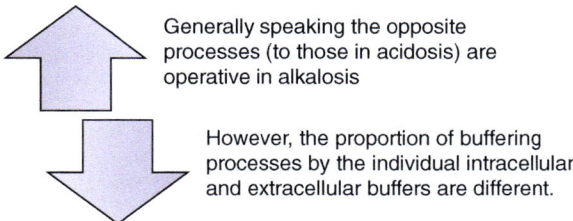

Pitts RF. Physiology of the kidney and body fluids. Chicago: Year Book; 1974. Chapter 11.
Rose B, Post T. Buffers-II, In: www.utd.com. Last updated: Oct 6, 2010. Last accessed: 13 May 2012.

4.16   Site Buffering

Just under 60 % of all buffering occurs *intra*cellularly; over 40 % of all buffering occurs *extra*cellularly.

Respiratory acid is mostly buffered intracellularly. CO_2 easily diffusible into ICF and is mostly buffered intracellularly; CO_2 cannot be buffered extracellularly where the bicarbonate buffer system is the dominant buffer (the bicarbonate buffer system cannot buffer one of its own components, CO_2).	**Buffering in respiratory acidosis**	Most of the buffering (approximately 99 %*) occurs in the ICF.
	Buffering in respiratory alkalosis	Most of the buffering (approximately 97 %*) occurs in the ICF.

Metabolic acid is mostly buffered extracellularly.	**Buffering in metabolic acidosis**	Approximately 40 % of the buffering occurs in the ECF.
		Approximately 60 % of the buffering occurs in the ICF.
	Buffering in metabolic alkalosis	Approximately 70 % of the buffering occurs in the ECF.
		Approximately 30 % of the buffering occurs in the ICF.

Brandis K. Acid-base pHysiology. www.anaesthesiaMCQ.com. Last accessed 6 June 2012.

Madias NE, Cohen JJ. Acid-base chemistry and buffering. In: Cohen JJ, Kassirer JP, editors. Acid-base. Boston: Little, Brown; 1982.

4.17 Isohydric Principle

According to the isohydric principle all the buffer systems within the body exist in equilibrium with each other; therefore analysis of any one buffer systems of the body mirrors the state of all the other buffer systems.

The non-bicarbonate buffer system	The bicarbonate buffer system		
The non bicarbonate buffer system is in reality a conglomeration of several different buffer systems.	The bicarbonate buffer system is the most convenient to measure. Its measurement effectively provides quantitative information about the other buffer systems of the body.		
Because of its inhomogeneity, it is difficult to measure.	**pH**	**CO_2**	**HCO_3^-**
	Measured by the ABG machine.	*Measured* by the ABG machine	*Calculated* from Henderson-Hasselbach equation.

4

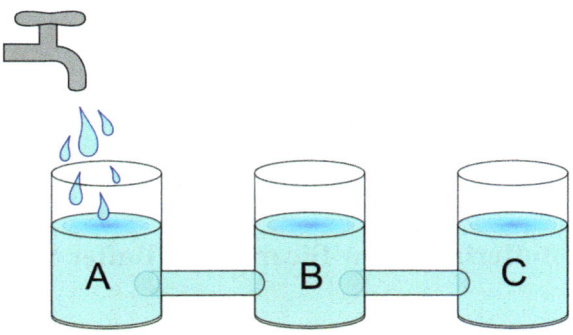

A non-bicarbonic acid that is added to the blood can be converted into carbonic acid and then eliminated through the lungs as CO_2.

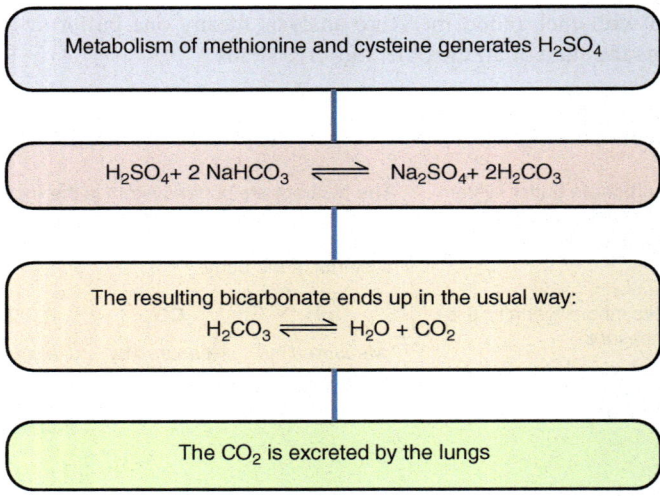

4

4.18   Base–Buffering by the Bicarbonate Buffer System

The bicarbonate buffer system is equally efficient at handling extraneous bases. In respect of added sodium hydroxide:

$NaOH + CO_2 \rightleftharpoons NaCO_3$

Or more properly,

$NaOH + H_2CO_3 \rightleftharpoons NaHCO_3 + H_2O$

Pitts RF. Physiology of the kidney and body fluids. Chicago: Year Book; 1974. Chapter 11.

Rose B, Post T. Buffers-II. In: www.utd.com. Last updated Oct 6, 2010. Last accessed 13 May 2012.

4.19   Bone Buffering

Bone has a large surface area and is an extremely efficient buffer.

The adult skeleton holds approximately 25,000 mEq of alkali: all this can provide an enormous buffering reserve for acid loads. Bone is also the major reservoir for CO_2; it contains 5/6 of the body's pool of CO_2, in the form of:

Bicarbonates (a hydration shell retains the bicarbonate in an easily exchangeable form) and

Carbonates (CO3).

Bone buffering is relatively slow, but its buffer reserve is vast.

4

Acute metabolic acidosis	Chronic metabolic acidosis	
As much as 40 % of all buffering is by bone.	The degree of buffering by bone is even greater, and may actually result in its dissolution (skeletal muscle breakdown and muscular wasting may also occur). In end-stage renal disease, the kidneys are ineffecient at excreting acids.	

Release of Na^+ and K^+	Release of Ca^{++}: demineralization	Osteoclastic resorption
Na^+ and K^+ are exchanged for H^+	As the acidosis gets established, Ca^{++} begins to participate in the ion exchange. Both osteoclastic and osteoblastic processes involving viable bone cells, occur. The Ca^{++} release is not merely on account of physicochemical buffering.	Osteoclastic resorption occurs in long-standing metabolic acidosis (uremia, renal tubular acidosis).

Chabala JM, Levi-Setti R, Bushinsky DA. Alterations in surface ion composition of cultured bone during metabolic, but not respiratory, acidosis. Am J Physiol. 1991;261:F76.

Green J, Kleeman CR. Role of bone in regulation of systemic acid-base balance. Kidney Int. 1991;39:9.

4.20   Role of the Liver in Acid–Base Homeostasis

The liver utilizes a large proportion of the blood supply of the body. It accounts for 20 % of the O_2 consumption of the entire body and contributes to 20 % of the total CO_2 production.

Substrate oxidation

Complete oxidation of fats and carbohydrates leading to CO_2 production.

Metabolism of organic acids

(i)   *Lactate metabolism*
About 1,500 mmol lactate is produced and consumed each day with virtually no net lactate production. Lactate is utilized for energy by some tissues.
Cori's cycle: Lactate is used as fuel for glucogenesis by the liver and kidney, converted to glucose and released into the blood. The glucose is taken up by peripheral tissues (e.g. exercising skeletal muscle) and converted to lactate.

(ii)   *Ketone metabolism*
Ketoacids (KAs) result from the incomplete oxidation of fats in hepatocyte mitochondria. Normally the daily output of KAs is quite small.
KAs are taken up by peripheral tissues (e.g. skeletal muscle) and oxidized, regenerating bicarbonate.

(iii)   *Amino acid metabolism*
Amino acid (AA) metabolism results in the production of:
- *Ammonium* from the NH_3^+ end of the AAs
- *Bicarbonate* from the COO^- end of the AAs
- *Fixed acids* from the side chains of the AAs

Metabolism of ammonium

Production of plasma proteins

Brandis K. Acid-base physiology. www.anaesthesiaMCQ.com. Last accessed 6 June 2012.

Cohen RD. Roles of the liver and kidney in acid-base regulation and its disorders. Br J Anaesth. 1991;67(2):154–64.

Chapter 5
pH

Contents

5

A. Hasan, *Handbook of Blood Gas/Acid-Base Interpretation*,
DOI 10.1007/978-1-4471-4315-4_5, © Springer-Verlag London 2013

5.1   Hydrogen Ion Activity

A distinction must be made between the actual concentration and the effective concentration of the hydrogen ion in solution.

Concentration	Effective concentration (Activity)
The number of particles in solution.	The number of particles that appear to be present in solution.

The activity **(a)** of a substance **(s)** can be represented by the following equation:

$$a = q\,c$$

where,

a = activity of the substance **s** in solution

q = the activity coefficient of the substance s

c = the concentration of the substance **s** in solution

In an ideal solution, the effective concentration should equal the actual concentration.

$a = c$

$a/c = q = 1$

Which is another way of saying that in an ideal solution, the activity coefficient should be 1.

In practice the activity coefficient of solutes is assumed to be one. The inaccuracies produced by this assumption are generally not clinically significant.

Brandis K. Acid-base physiology. www.anaesthesiaMCQ.com. Last accessed 6 June 2012.

5.2   Definitions of the Ad-hoc Committee of New York Academy of Sciences, 1965

Acidosis	An abnormal process or condition which would lower arterial pH if there were no secondary changes in response to the primary etiological factor.
Alkalosis	An abnormal process or condition which would raise arterial pH if there were no secondary changes in response to the primary etiological factor.
Simple (acid-base) disorders	Those (acid-base disorders) in which there is a single primary aetiological acid-base disorder.
Mixed (acid-base) disorders	Those (acid-base disorders) in which two or more *primary* aetiological disorders are present simultaneously.
Alkalemia	Arterial pH > 7.44 (i.e., H^+ < 36 nmol).
Acidemia	Arterial pH < 7.36 (i.e., H^+ > 44 nmol).

5

Winters RW. Terminology of acid-base disorders. Ann Intern Med 1965;63:873.

5.3   Acidosis and Alkalosis

5

Acidosis	Alkalosis
Acidosis is the process responsible for acidemia.	Alkalosis is the process responsible for alkalemia.
Acidosis leads to a fall in pH (acidemia) unless an opposing disturbance (alkalosis) is present or a compensatory mechanism is active.	Alkalosis leads to a rise in pH (alkalemia) unless an opposing disturbance (acidosis) is present or a compensatory mechanism is active.
Acidemia is therefore the usual (but not invariable) consequence of acidosis. Acidosis can exist without producing acidemia, but acidemia cannot exist in the absence of acidosis.	Alkalemia is therefore the usual (but not invariable) consequence of alkalosis. Alkalosis can exist without producing alkalemia, but alkalemia cannot exist in the absence of alkalosis.
Acidemia (as measured in the arterial blood) is the surrogate for acidosis, there being no practical way to measure tissue pH.	Alkalemia (as measured in the arterial blood) is the surrogate for alkalosis, there being no practical way to measure tissue pH.

Winters RW. Terminology of acid-base disorders. Ann Intern Med 1965;63:873.

5.4   The Law of Mass Action

According to the law of mass action, the velocity of a reaction is proportional to the product of the concentration of its reactants.

For water, the law of mass action can be written as:

$$H_2O \rightleftharpoons [H^+] [OH^-]$$

V1 represents the velocity of the movement of this reaction to the right

$$V1 = k1 [H_2O]$$

(k1 being the rate constant of the reaction)

V2 represents the velocity of the movement of this reaction to the left

$$V2 = k2 [H^+] [OH^-]$$

(k2 being the rate constant of the reaction)

5

At equilibrium,

$$V1 = V2$$

Or,

$$k1 [H_2O] = k2 [H^+] [OH^-]$$

A third constant can now be derived for H_2O when it is 50 % dissociated into its component ions:

$$K = k1 / k2 = [H^+] [OH^-] / [H_2O]$$

Cohen JJ. Acid-base chemistry and buffering. In: Cohen JJ, Kassirer JP, editors. Acid/base. Boston: Little, Brown; 1982.

Rose BD, Post TW. Clinical physiology of acid-base and electrolyte disorders. 5th ed. New York: McGraw-Hill; 2001.

5.5   Dissociation Constants

The dissociation constant of an acid is represented by the letter kappa (k).

In respect of an acid, the law of mass action may be written as:

$$HA \rightleftharpoons [H^+][A^-]$$

Or,

$$Ka = [H^+][A^-]/[HA]$$

(Where Ka is the dissociation constant for that acid)

Ka, the dissociation constant

Ka, the dissociation constant is different for each acid system. For all practical purposes, the *value of Ka is always the same for a particular acid* in a system (though it does change a little with temperature, the concentration of the solute and H^+).

The dissociation constant determines just how much of the acid dissociates in a system; it is a measure of the strength of an acid.

Stronger acids have larger dissociation constants	**Weaker acids have smaller dissociation constants**
They tend to dissociate more completely in solution.	They tend to dissociate relatively less in solution.

Gennari FJ, Cohen JJ, Kassirer JP. Measurement of acid-base status. In: Cohen JJ, Kassirer JP, editors. Acid/base. Boston: Little, Brown; 1982.

Kruse JA, Hukku P, Carlson RW. Relationship between apparent dissociation constant of blood carbonic acid and disease severity. J Lab Clin Med 1989; 114:568.

5.6   pK

pK is the negative log of the dissociation constant.

pK is the pH of the solution when an acid within that solution is 50 % dissociated.

The closer the pK of a buffer is to the pH of the system in which it operates, the more powerful will its effect be.

5

A buffer solution (see Sect. 4.4) is one that minimizes the changes in the hydrogen ion concentration that are produced by chemical reactions.

5.7   The Buffering Capacity of Acids

5.7.1   Buffering Power

A buffer is a mixture of an undissociated weak acid (HA) and its buffer base (A).
A weak acid is a better buffer than a strong acid.

Strong acid (e.g. NaCl)	Weak acid (e.g. Phosphate)
A strong acid has a higher dissociation constant and a lower pK.	A weak acid has a lower dissociation constant and a higher pK.
A strong acid dissociates to a greater degree. Within the usual range of pH in the body, a strong acid exists in a nearly fully dissociated state.	**A weak acid dissociates to a lesser degree.** Within the usual range of pH in the body, a weak acid exists in an only partly dissociated state.
Being dissociated to a greater degree, a strong acid has a poor affinity for the hydrogen ion. Strong acids are therefore poor at buffering hydrogen ions.	**Being poorly dissociated, a weak acid has a relatively strong affinity for the hydrogen ion.** Weak acids are therefore better at "absorbing" any surplus of hydrogen ions.
Strong acids make poor buffers.	$[HPO_4^-] + [H^+] \longleftarrow H_2PO_4$ Since the reaction is strongly driven to the right, a surplus of H^+ is well "absorbed". A surplus of H^+ drives the reaction to the right; a loss of H^+ drives it to the left. **Weak acids make good buffers.**

5.8 The Modified Henderson-Hasselbach Equation

The law of mass action as applied to the carbonic acid system:

The following equation represents the dissociation of carbonic acid:	The following equation represents the reaction between H_2O and CO_2 to reversibly form H_2CO_3:
$$H_2CO_3 \rightleftharpoons [H^+] + [HCO_3^-]$$ Applying the law of mass action, $$[H_2CO_3]\ Ka \rightleftharpoons [H^+]\ [HCO_3^-]$$ Or, $$Ka = [H^+]\ [HCO_3^-]\ /[H_2CO_3]$$ (Where, Ka is the dissociation constant of carbonic acid). Rearranging, $$Ka/[H^+] = [HCO_3^-]/H_2CO_3$$	$$H_2CO_3 \rightleftharpoons H_2O + CO_2$$
$Ka = 2.72 \times 10^{-4}$ H^+ concentration $= 40 \times 10^{-9}$ *Inserting the above values into the equation,* $$[HCO_3^-]/[H_2CO_3]$$ $$= [2.72 \times 10^{-4}]/[40 \times 10^{-9}]$$ $$= 6,800$$ i.e. **6,800 molecules of HCO_3^- are present for every molecule of H_2CO_3.**	For the above reaction it can be shown that the dissociation constant is far to the right. **340 molecules of CO_2 are present for every molecule of H_2CO_3.**

Putting the two equations together,

$$[H^+]\ [HCO_3] \rightleftharpoons [H_2CO_3]\ k1 \rightleftharpoons [H_2O]\ [CO_2]\ k2$$

Only 1 molecule of H_2CO_3 is present for 6,800 molecules of HCO_3,
Only 1 molecule of H_2CO_3 is present for 340 molecules of CO_2.
Since it is present in relatively low concentrations, H_2CO_3 can be disregarded.
H_2O is being 'constant' can also be disregarded.

The equation now becomes:

$[H^+] [HCO_3] \rightleftharpoons [CO_2]$ K'a (where K'a is a new constant)
Rearranging,

$$K'a = [H^+] [HCO_3]/[CO_2]$$

Or:

$$[H^+] = K'a [CO_2]/[HCO_3]$$

At 37 °C (normal body temperature), K'a = 800 x 10 (9) nmol/L pKa = 6.10
Since

$$[H^+] = K'a [CO_2]/[HCO_3],$$
$$[H^+] = 800 [CO_2]/[HCO_3]$$

Multiplying CO_2 by 0.03 (its solubility constant in the plasma)

$$[H^+] = 800 \times 0.03/[HCO_3]$$

The equation now becomes:

$$[H^+] = 24 \times [CO_2]/[HCO_3]$$

This is Kassirer and Bleich modification* of the Henderson-Hasselbach equation.

*Narins RG, Emmet M. Simple and mixed acid-base disorders: a practical approach. Medicine (Baltimore) 1980; 59:161–87.

Brandis K. Acid-base physiology. www.anaesthesiaMCQ.com. Last accessed 6 June 2012.

Hills AG. pH and the Henderson-Hasselbalch equation. Am J Med 1973; 55:131.

Kassirer JP. Serious acid-base disorders. N Engl J Med 1974; 291:773.

Kassirer JP, Bleich HL. Rapid estimation of plasma CO_2 from pH and total CO_2 content. N Engl J Med 1965; 272:1067.

5.9   The Difficulty in Handling Small Numbers

Relative to other ions in the body, the hydrogen ion exists in miniscule concentrations.

Concentration of some serum electrolytes:

Sodium:
140 mmol/L

Porassium:
4 mmol/L

Concentration of hydrogen ion:
0.00004 mmol/L
To overcome the difficulty in handling such small numbers certain methods were introduced:

5

Sorensen, 1909
The pH

(see next section)

Campbell, 1862
The nanomole (nm)

1 nanomole = 10 (9) mole
1 nanomole = 1/1,000,000,000 mole

Severinghaus JW, Astrup P. History of blood as analysis. Int Anestn Clin 1987; 25:1–224.

5.10   The Puissance Hydrogen

In 1909 a Danish biochemist published a landmark paper in French. Soren Peter Sorensen observed that enzymatic activity produced tiny but measurable changes in the H^+ concentration.

Mathematically,

$$10 \text{ can be expressed as } 10^1$$

$$100 \text{ can be expressed as } 10^2$$

$$1000 \text{ can be expressed as } 10^3, \text{ (and so forth)}$$

Similarly,

$$1/10 \text{ can be expressed as } 10^{-1}$$

$$1/100 \text{ can be expressed as } 10^{-2}$$

$$1/1000 \text{ can be expressed as } 10^{-3} \text{ (and so forth).}$$

Sorensen 'used' these negative exponents to the base 10 to simplify handling of these numbers. He then discarded the negative sign from the power to which 10 was expressed, and called the number "pH", a short form for what he called the "Puissance hydrogen" or "Wasserstoffionenexponent" or simply the "Potenz" ie "Potential" of hydrogen. When the concentration of a substance is expressed as a negative power, the greater its negative power the lower the concentration is of that substance.

Sorensen used this method to express the concentration of the hydrogen ion. Thus, a hydrogen ion concentration of:

$$0.1 = pH\ 1$$

$$0.01 = pH\ 2$$

$$0.001 = pH\ 3 \text{ (and so forth).}$$

In Sorenson's new terminology, a molar solution of a strong acid having a hydrogen ion concentration of 0.01 (10^{-2}), had a pH of 2. Similarly, a hydrogen ion concentration of 0.00000001 (10^{-7}) was expressed as having a pH of 7.

Thus pH is the negative logarithm of the H^+ ion concentration in moles per liter of solution. It has no units: Kellum described it as the "dimensionless representation of the $[H^+]$".

The lower the concentration of the hydrogen ion in solution, the greater is the pH of that solution.

Kellum JA. Determinants of blood pH in health and disease. Crit Care. 2000; 4(1): 6–14.
Severinghaus JW, Astrup P. History of blood as analysis. Int Anestn Clin 1987; 25:1–224.

5.11 Why pH?

As mentioned above, the intent behind the use of the pH scale is to make the handling of very small numbers more convenient.

The hydrogen ion concentration of the blood under physiological conditions is about 0.00000004 mol/L (40 nano moles/L).

Compare this with, say, the plasma concentration of sodium which at 0.135–0.145 mol/L is some three million times greater.

5

Viewing things on a logarithmic scale, large changes in the H^+ concentration translate into only small changes in the pH.

A doubling of the H^+ concentration, (for instance, from 40 n mol/L to 80 n mol/L) causes a numeric fall in the pH only to the order of 0.3 (i.e., from 7.40 to 7.10).

In actual fact, a change in pH from 7.40 to 7.10 represents the addition of a huge amount (clinically speaking) of acid to the body.

The pH range 6.8–7.8 (corresponding to a H^+ ion concentration of 160–16 nmol/L) is generally considered to be the range of pH within which life can exist.

5.12   Relationship Between pH and H⁺

Analog scales have been developed to show the relationship between pH and H⁺ ion concentration. A rule of the thumb proposed by Kassirer and Bleich enables approximate conversion from one to the other.

Equivalent values of pH and H⁺		A pH of 7.40 corresponds to a H^+ ion concentration of 40 nEq/L. Using Kassirer and Bleich's rule, change in pH by every 0.01 unit represents a change in H^+ ion concentration by 1 nEq/L. Since pH and H^+ ion concentration are inversely related, a fall in pH from, for example, 7.40–7.38, represents a rise in the H^+ ion concentration from 40 to 42 nEq/L. A similar calculation can also be used for checking if the data are reliable (see Sect. 11.2).
pH	**[H⁺] (nanomoles/l)**	
6.8	158	
6.9	125	
7.0	100	
7.1	79	
7.2	63	
7.3	50	
7.4	40	
7.5	31	
7.6	25	
7.7	20	
7.8	15	

Kassirer JP, Bleich HL. Rapid estimation of plasma CO_2 from pH and total CO_2 content. N Engl J Med 1965; 272:1067.

5.13   Disadvantages of Using a Logarithmic Scale

On a logarithmic scale, a relatively small change in pH can reflect a large change in the H^+ ion concentration.

Because the scale is compressed at one end, changes of similar magnitude at different ends represent vastly different changes in the H^+ ion concentration.

A fall in pH from 7.0 to 7.1 represents an increase in the H^+ ion concentration by 20 nEq/L.	A fall in pH of the same magnitude from 7.6 to 7.5 represents a much smaller decrease in the H^+ ion concentration (by less than 10 nEq/L).

   In other words, as the blood becomes increasingly acidic, much smaller changes of pH are produced by the addition of relatively large quantities of H^+ ions. Intuitively relying on pH to gauge the H^+ ion concentration therefore could result in gross inaccuracies.

5

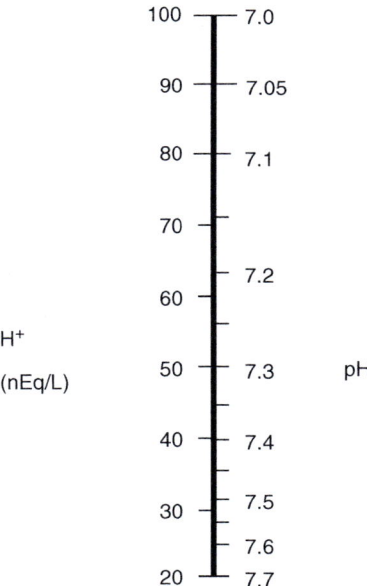

5.14 pH in Relation to pK

The capacity of a buffer to defend changes in the pH depends not only on its concentration in the system but also on the relationship between the pK of the system to the prevailing pH.

In respect of the bicarbonate buffer system which is the primary buffer system of the extracellular space:

When the concentration of bicarbonate equals the concentration of carbonic acid,

The ratio:

Bicarbonate/Carbonic acid

$$= 1/1$$

$$= 1$$

pH = pK + log
Bicarbonate/Carbonic acid
Since log 1 = 0
The pK of the system is 6.1,
pH = 6.1 + 0
pH = 6.1

The pH of the system equals its pK.
When the pH of the system equals its pK, the buffer systemis functioning at its maximum efficiency.

In vivo, the concentration of bicarbonate substantially exceeds the concentration of carbonic acid.
Bicarbonate = 27 mEq/L
Carbonic acid = 1.35 mEq/L
Ratio of Bicarbonate: Carbonic acid = 20

pH = 6.1 + log 27/1.35
pH = 6.1 + log 20
Since log 20 = 1.3
pH = 6.1 + 1.3
pH = 7.4

The pH of this system does not equal its pK.
The pH of this system is very different from the pK of the bicarbonate buffer system. This would make for a poor buffer system were it not for the continuous removal of CO_2 by the lungs (see Sects. 5.17 and 5.18).

5.15   Is the Carbonic Acid System an Ideal Buffer System?

Normal blood levels of HCO_3^- and CO_2:

HCO_3: 24 (range: 22–26) mEq/L

CO_2: 40 mmHg

i.e.,

0.03 x 40 = 1.2 mEq/L
(0.03 being the solubility coefficient of CO_2)

At the normal body pH of 7.4, the ratio of HCO_3:CO_2 = 24:1.2

$= 20$

An ideal buffer system should have a ratio of 1:1.

A HCO_3:CO_2 ratio of 20:1 would make for a rather poor buffer system were it not that both HCO_3:CO_2 can be independently regulated; the former by the kidneys and the latter by the lungs.

5

5.16   The Bicarbonate Buffer System Is Open Ended

The bicarbonate buffer system is open-ended in as much as both its components (HCO_3^- and CO_2) can be independently regulated by organ systems.

$$CO_2 \rightleftharpoons HCO_3$$

CO_2: regulated by the lungs

Central chemoreceptors are exquisitely sensitive to small changes in CO_2 (and therefore to the pH)

HCO_3: regulated by the kidneys

Generation of protons occurs in the renal tubular cells:

$$H_2O + CO_2 \rightleftharpoons H_2CO_3 \rightleftharpoons H^+ + HCO_3^-$$

Whenever the CO_2 increases for any reason,

this is accompanied by a prompt increase in alveolar ventilation

The protons [H^+] are secreted into the tubular lumen
In the tubular lumen the protons combine with NH_4, HPO_4 etc.

CO_2 washout occurs

As small as a 3 mmHg increase in $PaCO_2$ can result in a doubling of alveolar ventilation.

The bicarbonate generated by this reaction is absorbed into the circulation, which is effectively the excretion of one proton for every molecule of bicarbonate absorbed.

5.17   Importance of Alveolar Ventilation to the Bicarbonate Buffer System

$$[H^+] + [HCO_3^-] \rightleftharpoons H_2CO_3 ....(1)$$

$$H_2CO_3 \rightleftharpoons H_2O + CO_2 ....(2)$$

Within the physiological range of pH, the dissociation constant for reaction (2) ensures that the reaction is driven to the right. This means that there is always a large amount of CO_2 present in the plasma (for every molecule of H_2CO_3, 340 molecules of CO_2 are present).

CO_2 *(aqueous phase)*: PaCO$_2$= 1.2 mmol/L

The CO_2 present is in a dissolved state; the extent to which CO_2 remains dissolved in the plasma is proportional to its partial pressure, normally 40 mmHg.
Dissolved CO_2 = 40×0.03 = 1.2 mmol/L (where 0.03 is the solubility constant for CO_2).

CO_2 *(gas phase): PaCO$_2$ = 40 mm Hg*
The CO_2 in the blood is in equilibrium with alveolar CO_2.

CO_2 diffuses out of the capillary blood, through the 0.3 micron thick alveolo-capillary membrane, into the alveoli. Since CO_2 is highly diffusible across all biological membranes, the partial pressure of CO_2 in the alveolar air (**PACO$_2$**) approximates that in the pulmonary capillary blood (**PaCO$_2$**).

CO_2 *(alveolar air)*: PACO$_2$ = 40 mmHg
The disposal of CO_2 to the exterior by the lungs is the functional basis of the bicarbonate buffer system, which (in spite of a pK that differs substantially from the pH), is highly effective in disposing of the continually produced protons.

5

5.18   Difference Between the Bicarbonate and Non-bicarbonate Buffer Systems

Non-bicarbonate buffer systems

Alveolar ventilation plays no direct buffering role in the non-bicarbonate buffer systems. Non-bicarbonate buffer systems principally buffer changes in CO_2 since the bicarbonate is incapable of buffering a carbonic acid load (see also isohydric principle Sect. 4.17).

The carbonic acid buffer system

It cannot buffer any of its own constituents:

$$CO_2 + H_2O \rightleftharpoons H_2CO_3$$
$$H_2CO_3 \rightleftharpoons HCO_3^- + H^+$$
$$H^+ + HCO_3^- \rightleftharpoons H_2CO_3$$

A carbonic acid excess has to be buffered by *Intracellular buffers.*

Non-bicarbonate buffers as a measure of the pH:

As mentioned, the non-bicarbonate systems principally buffer changes in carbon-dioxide. It is possible to arrive at the H^+ concentration or the pH of the blood by measuring the status of the non-bicarbonate buffer system. However, since the non-bicarbonate buffer system is in reality a conglomeration of several buffer systems, measurement is complex. It is far less complicated to rather measure the constituents of the bicarbonate buffer system in order to calculate the pH.

5.19   Measuring and Calculated Bicarbonate

The measured bicarbonate is not the same as the calculated bicarbonate. The bicarbonate level of the blood can be estimated in different ways:

Calculated bicarbonate	Measured bicarbonate
Bicarbonate is calculated from the blood gas sample	Bicarbonate is chemically estimated from the venous blood sample (e.g., from a serum electrolyte sample). It is an estimate of not only the venous HCO_3^- but all the acid-labile forms of CO_2. For this reason the measured HCO_3^- is always 2-3 mEq/L greater than the calculated HCO_3^- (See total CO_2, Sect. 9.19).

5

When there is a discrepancy between the measured and calculated bicarbonate:

The venous HCO_3^- is actually the total CO_2 content, which is a measure of all the acid-labile forms of carbon dioxide (plasma HCO_3^- constitutes about 95 % of this). The measured venous HCO_3^- (total CO_2 content) exceeds the calculated arterial HCO_3^- by 2–3 mEq/L.

The pK of the bicarbonate buffer system may not be 6.1 in the critically ill; the calculated bicarbonate may therefore be erroneous.

Blood drawing by applying a tourniquet can result in a local lactic acidosis; this will lower the bicarbonate leading to falsely low measured bicarbonate.

Usually, venous HCO_3^- samples are processed later than arterial blood gas samples. If the standing time of the venous sample is prolonged, its bicarbonate content may become altered.

Chapter 6
Acidosis and Alkalosis

Contents

6

A. Hasan, *Handbook of Blood Gas/Acid-Base Interpretation*,
DOI 10.1007/978-1-4471-4315-4_6, © Springer-Verlag London 2013

6.1   Compensation

The body attempts to maintain its pH when confronted with acid-base. The compensatory processes are different for respiratory and renal disturbances. It is believed that in simple acid-base disorders, it is the change in pH (and not the change in CO_2 or HCO_3) produced by the inciting primary disturbance that is the stimulus for compensation.

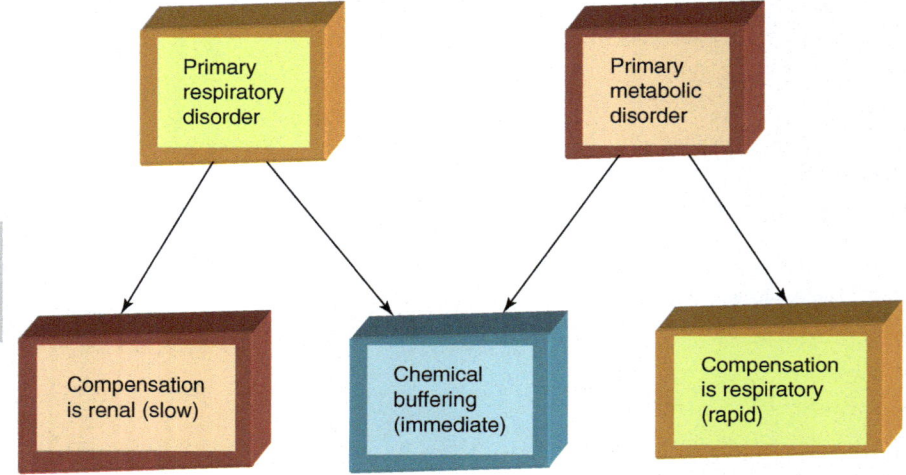

Lennon EJ, Lemann J Jr. pH- is it defensible? Ann Intern Med. 1966;65:1151.

McCurdy DK. Mixed metabolic and respiratory acid base disturbances: diagnosis and treatment. Chest. 1972;63:355S.

6.2   Coexistence of Acid Base Disorders

Frequently, two (sometimes three) acid-base disorders occur simultaneously.

Coexistence of multiple acid base disorders

Two respiratory disorders cannot coexist:
The lungs cannot simultaneously retain and excrete CO_2!

Other combinations of the four (simple) acid base disorders are possible:

Two metabolic disorders can occur together.

One metabolic disorder can occur together with a single respiratory disturbance.

Two metabolic disorders can occur together with a single respiratory disturbance.

6

McCurdy DK. Mixed metabolic and respiratory acid base disturbances: diagnosis and treatment. Chest. 1972;63:355S.

Narins RG, Emmet M. Simple and mixed acid-base disorders: a practical approach. Medicine (Baltimore). 1980;59:161.

6.3   Conditions in Which pH Can Be Normal

Normal pH is possible under three circumstances:

No acid-base disturbance exists	CO_2 and HCO_3^- are both in the normal range.	
A single acid-base disturbance is being fully compensated	**CO_2 and HCO_3^- are both low:**	Compensated respiratory alkalosis
	Either of the two following disturbances is present:	Compensated metabolic acidosis
	CO_2 and HCO_3^- are both high:	Compensated respiratory acidosis
	Either of the two following disturbances is present:	Compensated metabolic alkalosis
At least two acid-base disorders co-exist (a primary acidemia is being balanced out by a primary alkalemia).	**CO_2 and HCO_3^- are both high**	A primary respiratory acidosis + a primary metabolic alkalosis
	CO_2 and HCO_3^- are both low	A primary respiratory alkalosis + a primary metabolic acidosis
	CO_2 and HCO_3^- are both normal	A primary metabolic acidosis is offsetting a primary metabolic alkalosis.

6.4   The Acid Base Map

The acid base map shows the relationship between pH (or H$^+$), PaCO$_2$ and HCO$_3^-$. Shown on the map are 95 % confidence bands for the various acid-base disorders. When blood gas values are plotted on the map it becomes easy to rapidly diagnose single or mixed acid-base disturbances.

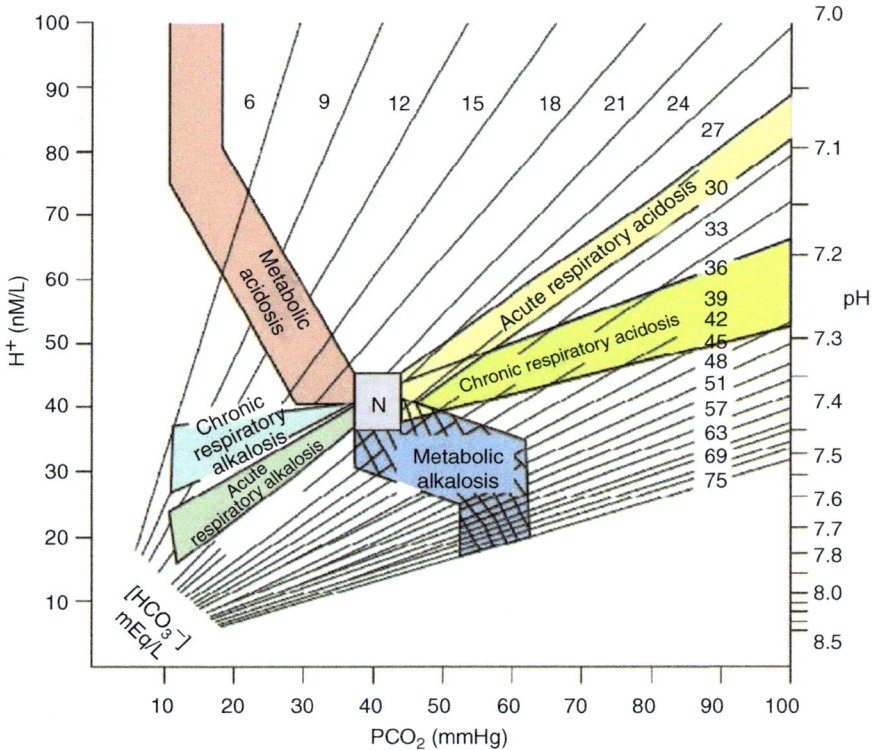

Goldberg M, Green SB, Moss ML, et al. Computer based instruction and diagnosis of acid-base disorders: a systematic approach. JAMA. 1973;223:269–75.

Chapter 7
Respiratory Acidosis

Contents

7

A. Hasan, *Handbook of Blood Gas/Acid-Base Interpretation*,
DOI 10.1007/978-1-4471-4315-4_7, © Springer-Verlag London 2013

7.1 Respiratory Failure

Although four types of respiratory failure have been described, it is usual to classify respiratory failure into Type-1 and Type-2: the latter is associated with hypoventilation and respiratory acidosis (see Sect. 7.2).

Respiratory failure			
Type 1 (Hypoxemic respiratory failure)	**Type 2 (Hypercapnic respiratory failure)**	**Type 3 (Per-operative respiratory failure)**	**Type 4 (Shock with hypo perfusion)**
PaO_2 is low ($PaO_2 < 50$ mmHg) CO_2 is not elevated ($PaCO_2 < 60$ mmHg) See Sect. 1.25	PaO_2 is low ($PaO_2 < 50$ mmHg) CO_2 is elevated ($PaCO_2 > 60$ mmHg) See Sect. 1.26	FRC falls below closing volume as a result of atelectasis. *Contributing factors:* Supine posture General anesthesia Depressed cough reflex Splinting due to pain	The proportion of the cardiac output to the respiratory muscles rises by as much as ten-fold when the work of breathing is high; this can seriously impair coronary perfusion during shock.

7

7.2   The Causes of Respiratory Acidosis

In terms of CO_2 production and excretion, alveolar hypoventilation is the major mechanism for hypercarbia (See Sects. 1.34 and 1.35). Quite often however, increase in dead space is an important mechanism (Sect. 1.30).

Causes of acute hypercapnia		Causes of chronic hypercapnia
Central depression of respiratory drive *Drugs* Sedatives, opiates, anaesthetic agents *CNS lesions* CNS trauma, strokes, encephalitis *Neuromuscular* Spinal cord lesions or trauma (at or above level of C4) High central neural blockade Tetanus Poliomyelitis Amyotrophic lateral sclerosis Myasthenia gravis Organophosphate poisoning Botulism Muscular relaxants Dyselectreolytemias *Airways* Upper airway obstruction Aspiration Asthma or COPD	*Chest wall* Flail chest Diaphragmatic dysfunction: 　Paralysis 　Splinting 　Rupture *Pleura* Pneumothorax Rapid accumulation of a large pleural effusion *Lung parenchyma* Cardiogenic pulmonary edema ARDS Pneumonia *Other* Circulatory shock Sepsis Malignant hyperthermia CO_2 insufflation into the body	*Central depression of respiratory drive* Primary alveolar hypoventilation *Neuromuscular* Chronic neuro-myopathies Poliomyelitis Dyselectreolytemias Malnutrition *Chest wall* Kyphoscoliosis Obesity Thoracoplasty *Pleura* Chronic large effusions *Lung parenchyma* Longstanding and severe ILD *Airways* Persistent asthma Severe COPD Bronchiectasis

7

7.3   Acute Respiratory Acidosis: Clinical Effects

A rapid decrease in alveolar ventilation is poorly tolerated by the body. Both acute hypercapnia and acute hypoxemia can be extremely damaging. However, surprising degrees of hypercapnia and hypoxemia can be tolerated by the body when chronic.

Acute	Chronic
• Poorly tolerated: can result in dangerous fluxes in the acid base status of the body	• Relatively well tolerated: due to compensatory mechanisms; patients may remain asymptomatic with very high $PaCO_2$ levels (e.g., over 100 mmHg)

Most clinical manifestations of acute hypercapnia are to do with the central nervous system.

Clinical features of Hypercapnia	
Sympahetic stimulation	Tachycardia, arrythmias Sweating Reflex peripheral vasoconstriction
Peripheral vasodilatation (a direct effect of hypercapnia)	Headaches, hypotension (if hypercapnia is severe).
Central depression (occurs at very high CO_2 levels)	Drowsiness, flaps, coma.
Decreased diaphragmatic contractility & endurance	Respiratory muscle fatigue.
Cerebral vasodilatation (results in increased intracranial pressure)	Confusion, headache; papilledema, loss of consciousness (if severe); hyperventilation.

Alberti E, Hoyer S, Hamer J, Stoeckel H, Packschiess P, Weinhardt F. The effect of carbon dioxide on cerebral blood flow and cerebral metabolism in dogs. Br J Anaesth. 1975;47:941–7.

Kilburn KH. Neurologic manifestations of respiratory failure. Arch Intern Med. 1965;116:409–15.

Neff TA, Petty TL. Tolerance and survival in severe chronic hypercapnia. Arch Intern Med. 1972;129:591–6.

Smith RB, Aass AA, Nemoto EM. Intraocular and intracranial pressure during respiratory alkalosis and acidosis. Br J Anaesth. 1981;53:967–72.

7.4   Effect of Acute Respiratory Acidosis on the Oxy-hemoglobin Dissociation Curve

Acute hypercapnia can transiently shift the oxy-hemoglobin dissociation curve to the right.

| Acute hyper-capnia | The oxy-Hb dissociation curve shifts rightwards | When hypercapnia becomes chronic, 2,3 DPG levels within RBC fall | The oxy-Hb dissociation curve shifts back towards normal |

Respiratory acidosis can decrease glucose uptake in peripheral tissues, and inhibit anaerobic glycolysis. When severe hypoxia is present, energy requirements can be critically compromised.

Bellingham AJ, Detter JC, Lenfant C. Regulatory mechanisms of hemoglobin oxygen affinity in acidosis and alkalosis. J Clin Invest. 1971;50:700–6.

Oski FA, Gottlieb AJ, Delivoria-Papadopoulos M, Miller WW. Red-cell 2, 3-diphosphoglycerate levels in subjects with chronic hypoxemia. N Engl J Med. 1969;280:1165–6.

7.5   Buffers in Acute Respiratory Acidosis

The bicarbonate buffer system, quantitatively the most important buffer system in the body, cannot buffer changes produced by alterations in CO_2, one of its own components. CO_2 changes are buffered therefore by non-bicarbonate buffer systems.

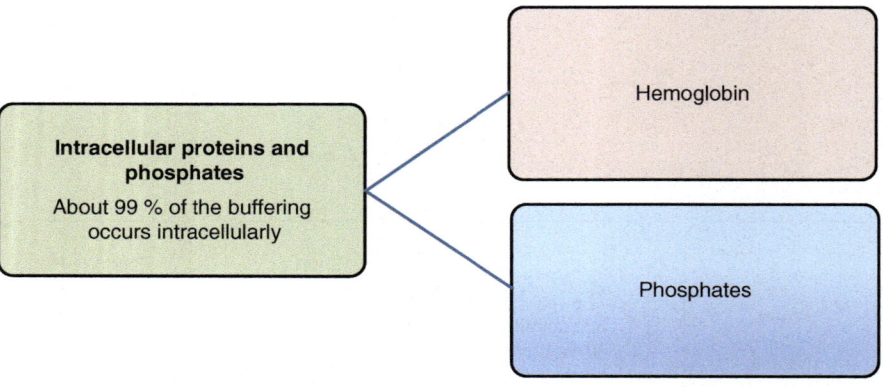

7.6   Respiratory Acidosis: Mechanisms for Compensation

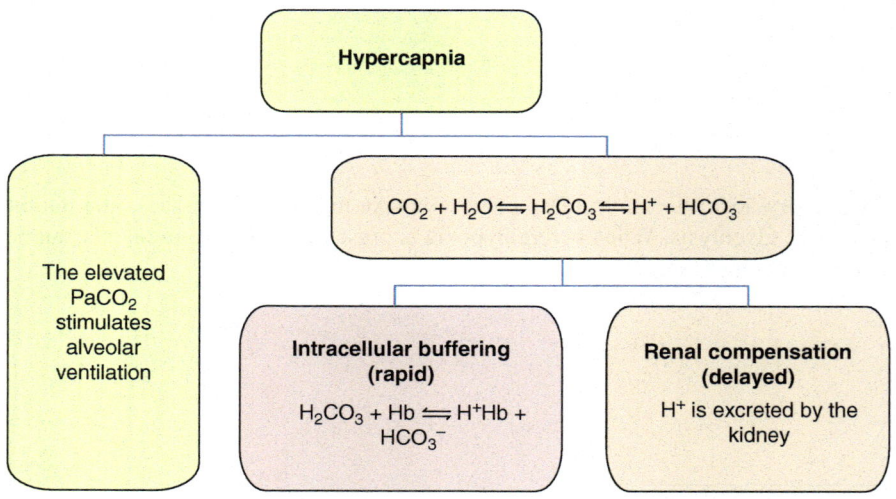

Brackett NC Jr, Wingo CF, Mureb O, et al. Acid-base response to chronic hypercapnia in man. New Eng J Med. 1969;280:124–30.

7.7 Compensation for Respiratory Acidosis

The following formulae are used to determine the extent of the compensatory processes, or if a second primary acid-base disorder is present.

Acute respiratory acidosis (<24 h)	Chronic respiratory acidosis (>24 h)
• $\Delta\downarrow*pH = 0.008 \times \Delta\uparrow PaCO_2$	• $\Delta\downarrow pH = 0.003 \times \Delta\uparrow PaCO_2$
• $\Delta H^+ = 0.8 \times \Delta PaCO_2$	• $\Delta H^+ = 0.3 \times \Delta PaCO_2$
• HCO_3^- increases by up to 0.1 mEq/L for every mmHg rise in CO_2	• HCO_3^- increases by up to 0.4 mEq/L for every mmHg rise in CO_2
• $H^+ = (0.8 \times PaCO_2) + 8$	• $H^+ = (0.3 \times PaCO_2) + 27$

Limits of compensation for respiratory acidosis
• The process of compensation is generally complete within 2 – 4 days.
• The bicarbonate is increased to a maximum of 45 mmol/L; a bicarbonate level in excess of this may imply a coexistent primary metabolic alkalosis.

7

$*\Delta = $ Change in; $\Delta\downarrow = $ Fall in; $\Delta\uparrow = $ Rise in

Smith RM. In: Bordow RA, Ries AL, Morris TA, editors. Manual of clinical problems in pulmonary medicine. 6th ed. Philadelphia: Lippincott Williams and Wilkins; 2005.

7.8   Post-hypercapnic Metabolic Alkalosis

Although the immediate event is hyperventilation with CO_2 washout, the blood gas reflects metabolic alkalosis.

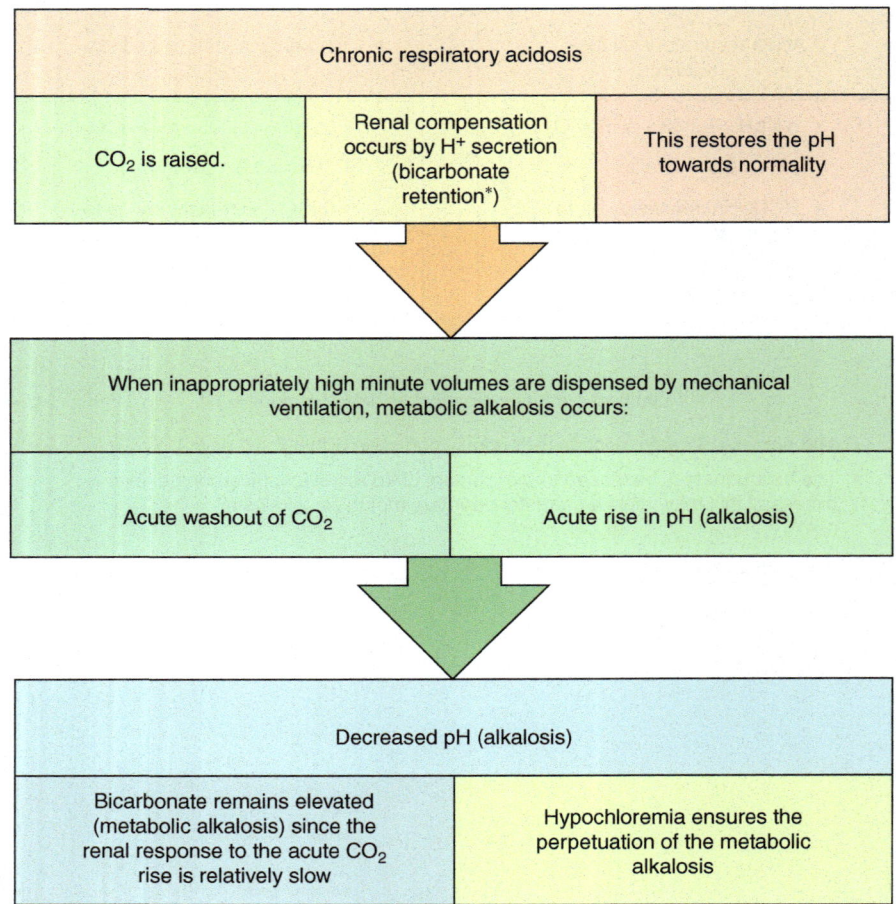

*The chronic elevation of bicarbonate results in chloride loss

Schwartz WB, Hays RM, Polak A, Haynie G. Effects of chronic hypercapnia on electrolyte and acid-base equilibrium. II. Recovery with special reference to the influence of chloride intake. J Clin Invest. 1961;40:1238.

7.9   Acute on Chronic Respiratory Acidosis

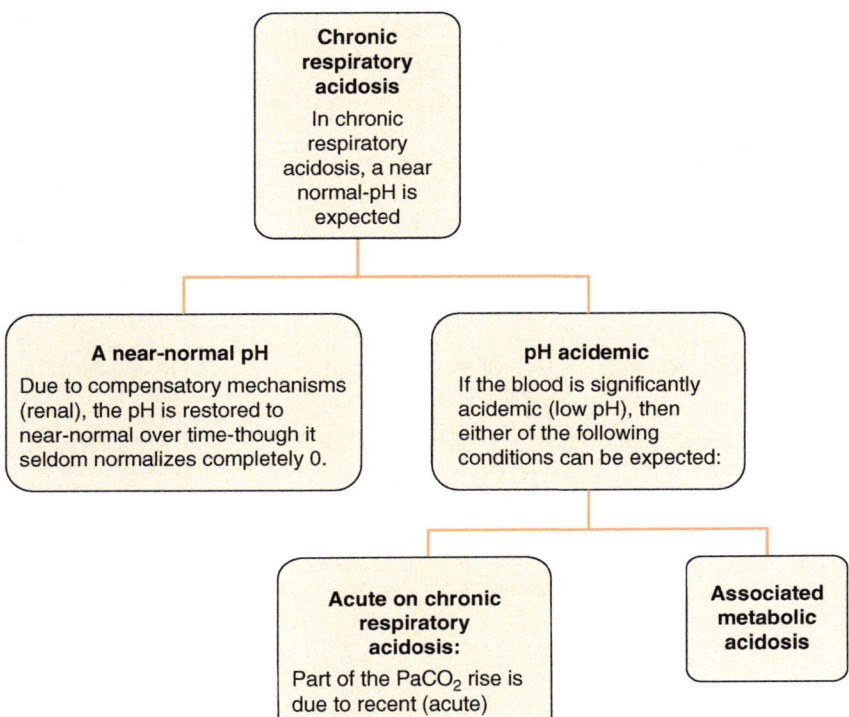

7.10   Respiratory Acidosis: Acute or Chronic?

Using the modified Henderson Hasselbach equation,

$$H^+ = 24(PaCO_2/HCO_3^-)$$

(H^+ = normally 40 nmol/L) The ratio $\Delta H^+/\Delta CO_2$ differs in each of the following conditions:

Acute respiratory acidosis:	Acute-on-chronic respirtory acidosis	Chronic respiratory acidosis:
$\Delta H^+/\Delta CO_2$ = >0.7	$\Delta H^+/\Delta CO_2$ = 0.3–0.7	$\Delta H^+/\Delta CO_2$ = <0.3
Case example: *PaCO_2 = 80 mmHg;* *HCO_3^- = 20 mEq/L* **H^+ = 24 (PaCO_2/HCO_3^-)** *Substituting,* H^+ = 24 (80/20) H^+ = 96 *Normal H^+ = 40;* *Normal PaCO_2 = 40* $\Delta H^+ / \Delta CO_2$ = (96–40) / (80–40) $\Delta H^+ / \Delta CO_2$ =1.4 *i.e, the value falls above 0.7*	**Case example:** *PaCO_2 = 90 mmHg;* *HCO_3^- = 30 mEq/L* **H^+ = 24 (PaCO_2/HCO_3^-)** *Substituting,* H^+ = 24 (90/30) H^+ = 72 *Normal H^+ = 40;* *Normal PaCO_2 = 40* $\Delta H^+ / \Delta CO_2$ = (72–40) / (90–40) $\Delta H^+ / \Delta CO_2$ = 0.44 *i.e, the value falls between 0.3 and 0.7*	**Case example:** *PaCO_2 = 90 mmHg;* *HCO_3^- = 45 mEq/L* **H_+ = 24 (PaCO_2/HCO_3^-)** Substituting, H^+ =24 (90/45) H^+ = 48 *Normal H^+ = 40;* *Normal PaCO_2 = 40* $\Delta H^+ / \Delta CO_2$ =(48–40) / (90–40) $\Delta H^+ / \Delta CO_2$ = 0.16 *i.e, the value falls below 0.3*

7

Demers RR, Irwin RS. Management of hypercapnic respiratory failure: a systematic approach. R Resp Care. 1979;24:328.

Chapter 8
Respiratory Alkalosis

Contents

8

A. Hasan, *Handbook of Blood Gas/Acid-Base Interpretation*,
DOI 10.1007/978-1-4471-4315-4_8, © Springer-Verlag London 2013

8.1 Respiratory Alkalosis

Unlike a metabolic alkalosis (where an additional mechanism is responsible for the maintenance of the acid-base disturbance), a respiratory alkalosis persists only as long as the inciting pathology is active.

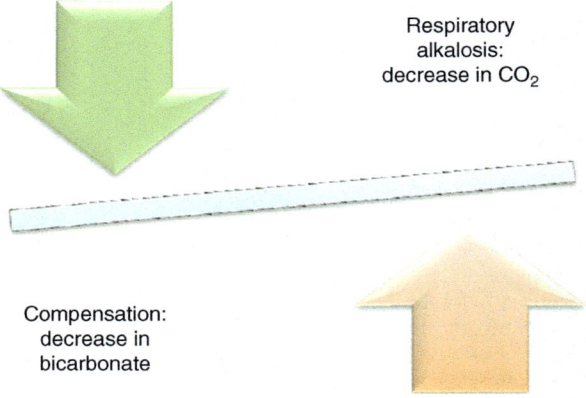

Respiratory alkalosis: decrease in CO_2

Compensation: decrease in bicarbonate

8

Rose BD, Post TW. Clinical physiology of acid-base and electrolyte disorders. 5th ed. New York: McGraw-Hill; 2001. p. 615–9.

8.2   Electrolyte Shifts in Acute Respiratory Alkalosis

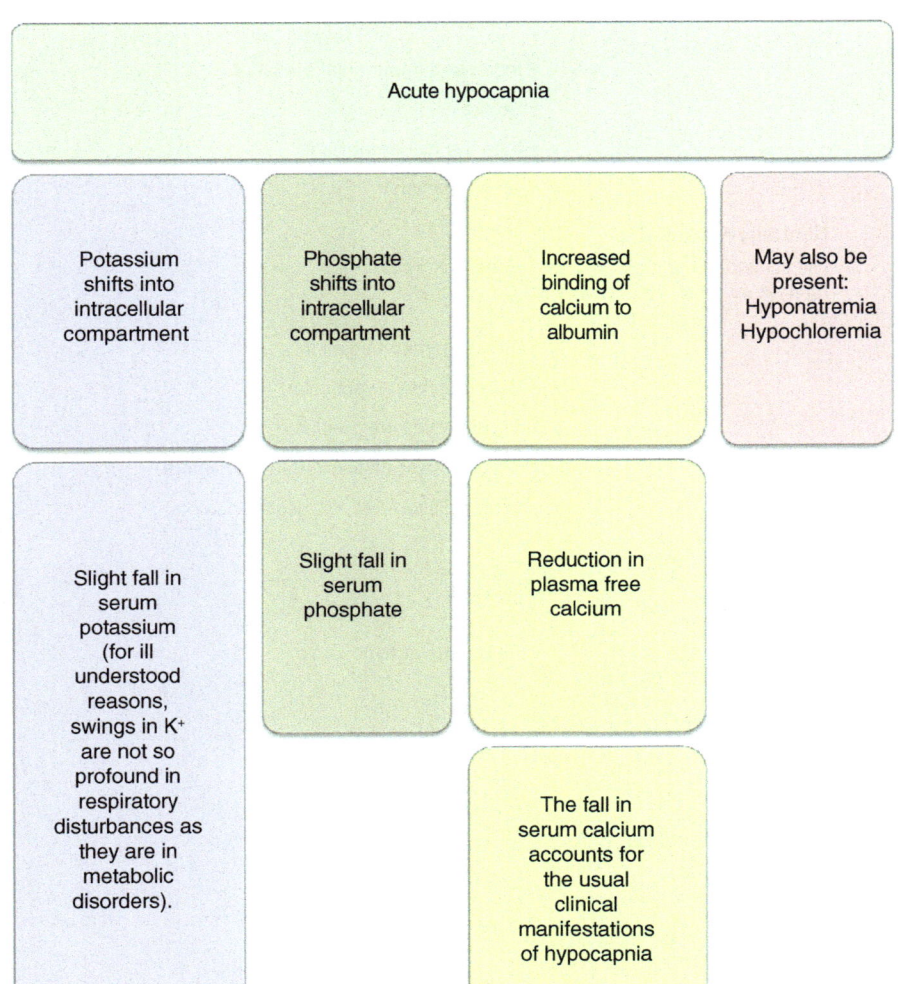

8

Karpf R, Caduff P, Wagdi P, Stäubli M, Hulter HN. Plasma potassium response to acute respiratory alkalosis. Kidney Int. 1995;47:217–24.

Wiseman AC, Linas S. Disorders of potassium and acid-base balance. Am J Kidney Dis. 2005; 45(5):941–9.

8.3   Causes of Respiratory Alkalosis

Centrally mediated

(By stimulation of the respiratory centre)

- Increased intracranial pressure
- Stroke
- Intracranial hemorrhage
- CNS infection
- Head injury
- Pontine tumours
- Pain
- Anxiety hyperventilation
- Voluntary hyperventilation
- Sepsis (cytokine mediated)
- Chronic Liver disease (toxin mediated)
- Drugs (Salicylates, progesterones etc)

Hypoxemic

(By stimulation of the peripheral chemoreceptors)

- All causes of hypoxemia

Pulmonary interstitial

(By stimulation of the intrapulmonary receptors)

- Pneumonia
- Asthma
- Pulmonary thromboembolism
- Pulmonary edema

Extrinsic

(Deliberate or iatrogenic)

- Excessive minute ventilation during mechanical ventilation

8

8.4   Miscellaneous Mechanisms of Respiratory Alkalosis

Hypotension	Tachypnea occurs due to excitation of peripheral chemoreceptors (directly, or in response to increases in catecholamine and angiotensin II levels). Later, hypoxemia and acidosis provide the stimulus to hyperventilate.
Central hyperventilation	Occurs in a variety of CNS conditions (Sect. 8.3) and results in several patterns of disordered breathing e.g., Central hyperventilation, Cheyne-Stoke's, and Biot's breathing.
Progesterone	During the luteal phase of the menstrual cycle, $PaCO_2$ levels drop by 3–8 mmHg. During the 3rd trimester of pregnancy, $PaCO_2$ stabilizes at 28–30 mmHg. Estrogen-progesterone combination pills induce more hyperventilation than progesterone alone, possibly because estrogens increase the expression of progesterone receptors.
Aminophylline	Aminophylline causes hyperventilation by a variety of mechanisms including adenosine receptor antagonism.
Salicylates	See below*. See also Sect. 9.35.
Hepatic failure	Possibly local cerebral hypoxia and increased levels of ammonia and progesterone play a part. The resultant hypocapnia partly restores cerebral autoregulation (at least in patients with *acute* liver failure), and may therefore be a protective response.
Septicemia	Fever, hypotension and hypoxemia can all stimulate respiration. The lipopolysaccharides of gram-negative bacilli may provoke tachypnea through additional mechanisms.
Heat exhaustion, heat stroke and cold exposure	Metabolic acidosis is the most common acid-base disorder in heat stroke, but severe respiratory alkalosis ($PaCO_2 \sim 20$ mmHg) can also be present. Near-drowning briefly produces hyperventilation following which ventilation falls and is driven by the metabolic status. In severe hypothermia, respiratory acidosis occurs as a consequence of CO_2 retention.
Pseudo-respiratory alkalosis	In severe circulatory failure or cardiac arrest, because of the sluggish circulation, pulmonary perfusion is reduced out of proportion to ventilation (high V/Q mismatch). Decreased delivery of CO_2 to the lungs precludes its effective excretion from the lungs, and CO_2 retention occurs. However, relative to the CO_2 that is delivered to the lungs, there is increased elimination (because of the increase in ventilation to perfusion ratio). Arterial eucapnia or even hypocapnia (*pseudorespiratory alkalosis*) can then prevail. The arteriovenous difference for pH, PO_2, and PCO_2 is substantially widened, but the relatively normal arterial O_2 values mask the severe tissue hypoxia. Central venous blood sampling usually reveals the true picture.

8

*Salicylic acid is a weak acid. Uncharged (protonated) molecules of salicylic acid easily cross the blood–brain barrier (BBB) and other cellular membranes. Alkalosis, by decreasing the concentration of uncharged particles, will prevent salicylate accumulation in the CSF. The respiratory alkalosis consequent to aspirin's actions on the medullary respiratory ionizes the salicylate particles and helps sequester them outside the BBB. Endotracheal intubation of patients in respiratory failure necessarily involves sedation and even paralysis, during which patients might suffer transient apnea. The resultant respiratory acidosis can generate large numbers of non-ionized particles which can now cross the BBB. This can prove fatal.

Adrogué HJ, Rashad MN, Gorin AB, Yacoub J, Madias NE. Arteriovenous acid-base disparity in circulatory failure: studies on mechanism. Am J Physiol. 1989a;257:F1087–93.

Adrogué HJ, Rashad MN, Gorin AB, Yacoub J, Madias NE. Assessing acid-base status in circulatory failure: difference between arterial and central venous blood. N Engl J Med. 1989b; 320:1312–6.

Bayliss DA, Millhorn DE. Central neural mechanisms of progesterone action: application to the respiratory system. J Appl Physiol. 1992;73:393–404.

Boyd AE, Beller GA. Heat exhaustion and respiratory alkalosis. Ann Intern Med. 1975;83:835.

Brashear RE. Hyperventilation syndrome. Lung. 1983;161:257–77.

Fadel HE, Northrop G, Misenheimer HR, Harp RJ. Normal pregnancy: a model of sustained respiratory alkalosis. J Perinat Med. 1979;7:195–201.

Gaudio R, Abramson N. Heat-induced hyperventilation. J Appl Physiol. 1968;25:742–6.

Grauberg PO. Human physiology under cold exposure. Arctic Med Res. 1991;50(Suppl 6):23–7.

Greenberg MI, Hendrickson RG, Hofman M. Deleterious effects of endotracheal intubation in salicylate poisoning. Ann Emerg Med. 2003;41:583.

Heymans C, Bouckaert JJ. Sinus caroticus and respiratory reflexes. J Physiol. 1930;69:254–73.

Pulm F. Hyperpnea, hyperventilation, and brain dysfunction. Ann Intern Med. 1972;76:328.

Ring T, Anderson PT, Knudesn F, Nielsen FB. Salicylate-induced hyperventilation. Lancet. 1985;1:1450.

Shugrue PJ, Lane MV, Merchenthaler I. Regulation of progesterone receptor messenger ribonucleic acid in the rat medical preoptic nucleus by estrogenic and antiestrogenic compounds. Endocrinology. 1997;138:5476–84.

Simmons DH, Nicoloff J, Guze LB. Hyperventilation and respiratoryalkalosis as sings of gram-negative bacteremia. JAMA. 1960;174:2196–9.

Stolbach AI, Hoffman RS, Nelson LS. Mechanical ventilation was associated with acidemia in a case series of salicylate-poisoned patients. Acad Emerg Med. 2008;15:866.

Strauss G, Hansen BA, Knudsen GM, Larsen FS. Hyperventilation restores cerebral blood flow autoregulation in patients with acute liver failure. J Hepatol. 1998;28:199–203.

Stround MA, Lambersten CJ, Ewing JH, Kough RH, Gould RA, Schmidt CF. The effects of aminophylline and meperidine alone and in combination on the respiratory response to carbon dioxide inhalation. J Pharmacol Exp Ther. 1955;114:461–74.

Takano N, Sakai A, Iida. Analysis of alveolar PCO_2 control during the menstrual cycle. Pfluegers Arch. 1981;390:56–62.

Winslow EJ, Loeb HS, Rahimtoola SH, Kamath S, Gunnar RM. Hemodynamic studies and results of therapy in 50 patients with bacteremic shock. Am J Med. 1973;54:421–32.

Yamamoto M, Nishimura M, Kobayashi S, Akiyama Y, Miyamoto K, Kawakami Y. Role of endogenous adenosine in hypoxic ventilatory response in humans: a study with dipyridamole. J Appl Physiol. 1994;76:196–203.

8.5   Compensation for Respiratory Alkalosis

The magnitude of the fall in the serum bicarbonate as a compensatory process is different in acute and chronic respiratory alkalosis.

Acute respiratory alkalosis (<12 h)	Chronic respiratory alkalosis (>12 h)
• $\Delta\uparrow pH = 0.01 \times \Delta\downarrow PaCO_2$*	• $\Delta\uparrow pH = 0.0003 \times \Delta\downarrow PaCO_2$
• $\Delta\downarrow H^+ = 0.75 \times \Delta\downarrow PaCO_2$	• $\Delta\downarrow H^+ = 0.3 \times \Delta\downarrow PaCO_2$
• HCO_3^- falls by up to 0.2 mEq/L for every mmHg fall in CO_2	• HCO_3^- falls by up to 0.5 mEq/L for every mmHg fall in CO_2
• $H^+ = (0.75 \times PaCO_2) + 10$	• $H^+ = (0.3 \times PaCO2) + 28$

Limits of compensation for respiratory alkalosis
• The process of compensation is generally complete within 7 to 10 days
• The serum bicarbonate can fall to as low as 12 mmol/L; a lower bicarbonate level may imply a coexistent primary metabolic acidosis.

*This relationship holds good for a $PaCO_2$ between 40 and 80 mmHg.

8

Krapf, R, Beeler, I, Hertner, D, Hulter, HN. Chronic respiratory alkalosis. The effect of sustained hyperventilation on renal regulation of acid-base equilibrium. N Engl J Med. 1991;324:1394.

Smith RM. In: Bordow RA, Ries AL, Morris TA, editors. Manual of clinical problems in pulmonary medicine. 6th ed. Philadelphia: Lippincott Williams and Wilkins; 2005.

8.6   Clinical Features of Acute Respiratory Alkalosis

Effects on regional blood flow in acute respiratory alkalosis

Decreased blood flow to:		Increased blood flow to:	
Heart, brain, kidney and skin		Skeletal muscle	

Central nervous system	Paresthesias, carpopedal spasm, circumoral numbness, muscle cramps, asterexis, confusion, loss of consciousness, generalized seizures (rare).		
Cardiovascular system	Arrythmias, coronary ischemia and variant angina, decreased cardiac contractility.		
Hemoglobin	Increased Hb affinity for O_2	Leftward shift in the ODC[*]	
	Increase in RBC 2,3,DPG levels	Rightward shift in ODC[*]	
Blood	Hemoconcentration (due to shift of plasma fluid out of the vascular compartment)		
Lungs	Increased O_2 uptake due to hypocapnia-induced Bohr effect (see Sects. 2.29 and 2.30).		
	Decreased O_2 release to the peripheral tissues. Decreased alveolar fluid resorption.		
Other	Electrolytes (see Sect. 8.2)		

*The overall effects are therefore unpredictable, but the position of the ODC may remain roughly unaltered

Ardissino D, De Servi S, Falcone C, Barberis P, Scuri PM, Previtali M, Specchia G, Montemartini C. Role of hypacapnic alkalosis in hyperventilation-induced coronary artery spasm in variant angina. Am J Cardiol. 1987;59:707–9.

Evans DW, Lum LC. Hyperventilation: an important cause of pseudoangina. Lancet. 1977;1:155–7.

Gotoh F, Meyer JS, Takagi Y. Cerebral effects of hyperventilation in man. Arch Neurol. 1965;12:410–23.

Kazmaier S, Weyland A, Buhre W, et al. Effect of respiratory alkalosis and acidosis on myocardial blood flow and metabolism in patients with coronary artery disease. Anesthesiology. 1998;89(4):831–7.

Kety SS, Schmidt CF. The effects of altered arterial tensions of carbon dioxide and oxygen on cerebral blood flow and cerebral oxygen consumption of normal young men. J Clin Invest. 1948;27:484–91.

Kirsch DB, Josefowicz RF. Neurologic complications of respiratory disease. Neurol Clin. 2002; 20(1):247–64.

Myrianthefs PM, Briva A, Lecuona E, et al. Hypocapnic but not metabolic alkalosis impairs alveolar fluid resorption. Am J Respir Crit Care Med. 2005;171(11):1267–71.

Stäubli M, Rohner F, Kammer P, Ziegler W, Straub PW. Plasma volume and proteins in voluntarily hyperventilation. J Appl Physiol. 1986;60:1549–53.

Stäubli M, Vogel F, Bärtsch P, Flückiger G, Ziegler WH. Hyperventilation induced changes in blood cell counts depend on hypocapnia. Eur J Appl Physiol. 1994;69:402–7.

Chapter 9
Metabolic Acidosis

Contents

9

A. Hasan, *Handbook of Blood Gas/Acid-Base Interpretation*,
DOI 10.1007/978-1-4471-4315-4_9, © Springer-Verlag London 2013

9

9.1   The Pathogenesis of Metabolic Acidosis

Simply stated, the pathogenesis of metabolic acidosis involves either a net gain of acid (hydrogen ions) or a net deficit of bicarbonate ions from the extracellular fluid.

Decreased acid-excretion by kidneys	• Renal failure • Type 1 (distal) RTA
Addition of strong acids to the body:	**Endogenous generation, e.g.:** • Ketoacids (in diabetic keto-acidosis) • Lactate (in lactic acidosis) **Exogenous administration, e.g.:** • Infusion of ammonium chloride
Loss of base (usually bicarbonate), from the body:	**Bicarbonate loss from the kidney:** • Type 2 RTA • Carbonic acid inhibitor use • Urinary ketoacid loss in DKA (ketoacids are the precursors of bicarbonate) **Bicarbonate loss from the bowel** • Diarrhea • Fistula of the small intestine

9

Mencken HL. Prejudices. Exeunt Omnes. New York: Borzoi; 1920. p. 180–93.

9.2   The pH, PCO_2 and Base Excess: Relationships

The approximate relationship between the pH, CO_2 and base excess can be summarized by the equation below:

$$PCO_2 \text{ 12 mmHg} \leftrightarrows pH \text{ 0.1} \leftrightarrows \text{Base excess 6 mEq/L}$$

According to this relationship, to produce a change in pH of 0.1 units, either the PCO_2 must change by 12 mmHg or the BE by 6 mEq/L

Now, consider the following hypothetical situations:

PCO_2 40 mmHg $\leftrightarrows$ pH 7.4 $\leftrightarrows$ BE–0

If now the PCO_2 were to rise to 52 and the BE to remain –0,
The rise of PCO_2 by 12 would cause the pH to fall by 0.1. The pH would now be 7.3 :

PCO_2 52 mmHg $\leftrightarrows$ pH 7.3 $\leftrightarrows$ BE– 0

Consider the following baseline again:

PCO_2 40 mmHg $\leftrightarrows$ pH 7.4 $\leftrightarrows$ BE –0

If now the PCO_2 were to fall to 28 and the BE to remain – 0,

The fall of PCO_2 by 12 would cause the pH to rise by 0.1. The pH would now be 7.5

PCO_2 28 mmHg $\leftrightarrows$ pH 7.5 $\leftrightarrows$ BE –0

PCO_2 40 mmHg $\leftrightarrows$ pH 7.4 $\leftrightarrows$ BE –0

In metabolic acidosis, if the BE were to fall to –6 and the PCO_2 to remain 40 mmHg, a fall in BE would cause a fall in pH of the order of 0.1 unit; the newph would fall to 7.3 :

PCO_2 40 mmHg $\leftrightarrows$ pH 7.3 $\leftrightarrows$ BE –6

Likewise, if the BE were to rise to +6 and the PCO_2 to remain at 40 mmHg, a rise in BE by 6 mEq/l would produce a rise in pH by 0.1 unit. The new pH would be 7.5 :

PCO_2 40 mmHg $\leftrightarrows$ pH 7.5 $\leftrightarrows$ BE +6

The impact on pH due to changes in both the PCO_2 and BE can also be predicted by the same equation:

$$PCO_2 \text{ 40 mmHg} \leftrightarrows pH \text{ 7.4} \leftrightarrows \text{BE –0}$$

What would be the pH with a PCO_2 of 52 and a BE of +6?

A rise in PCO_2 by 12 (from 40 to 52) mmHg would tend to lower the pH by 0.1. A rise in BE by 6 (from–0 to +6) mEq/L would tend to raise the pH by 0.1. As a result, the pH would remain unchanged at 7.4:

PCO_2 52 mmHg $\leftrightarrows$ pH 7.4 $\leftrightarrows$ BE +6

What would be the pH with a PCO_2 of 28 and a BE of +12?

A fall in PCO_2 by 12 (from 40 to 28) mmHg would tend to raise the pH by 0.1. A rise in BE by 12 (from–0 to +12) mEq/L would tend to raise the pH by 0.2. As a result, the net change in pH would be an in crease by 0.3 :

PCO_2 28 mmHg $\leftrightarrows$ pH 7.5 $\leftrightarrows$ BE +12

9

Grogono AW. Acid-Base Tutorial, http://www.acid-base.com/production.php. Last accessed 6 June 2012.

9.3 The Law of Electroneutrality and the Anion Gap

The Law of Electroneutrality states that the sum of all the anions should equal the sum of all the cations. In practice the measured anions are Sodium (Na^+) and Potassium (K^+), and the measured cations are Bicarbonate (HCO_3^-) and Chloride (Cl^-).

The anion gap is the difference between the unmeasured anions and the unmeasured cations.

$$Anion\ Gap = \left[Na^+\right] + \left[K^+\right] - \left[HCO_3^-\right] - \left[Cl^-\right]$$

The usual *measured ions are:*	Unmeasured ions:
The anion gap exists because some anions are not measured.	In wide anion gap metabolic acidoses (see later), there is a relative excess in the concentration of unmeasured anions.
It is "an artefact of measurement and not a physiological reality" (Martin)*	
In other words, if all ions were measurable, there would simply be no anion gap!	Although these anions are not directly measured, the increased H^+ in acidosis leads to consumption in the HCO_3^-.

Wide anion gap

The anion gap is widened because the sum of **measured** cations ($[Na^+] + [K^+]$) significantly exceeds the sum of the measured anions ($[HCO_3^-] + [Cl^-]$). This is because of the presence of an excess of *unmeasured anions* in the blood (see Sect. 9.4).

9

---

*Martin L. All you really need to know to interpret arterial blood gases. Philadelphia: Lippincott Williams and Wilkins; 1999.

Rose BD, Post TW. Clinical physiology of acid-base and electrolyte disorders. 5th ed. New York: McGraw-Hill; 2001. p. 583–8.

9.4   Electrolytes and the Anion Gap

By the Law of Electroneutrality: *Total cations − total anions = 0*

$$Na^+ + K^+ + \text{unmeasured cations} = Cl^- + HCO_3^- + \text{unmeasured anions}$$

Rearranging,

$$Na^+ + K^+ - Cl^- - HCO_3^- = \text{Unmeasured anions} - \text{Unmeasured cations}$$

$$\text{Anion gap} = \textit{unmeasured anions} - \textit{unmeasured cations}$$

The anion gap widens when unmeasured anions are increased or unmeasured cations are decreased.

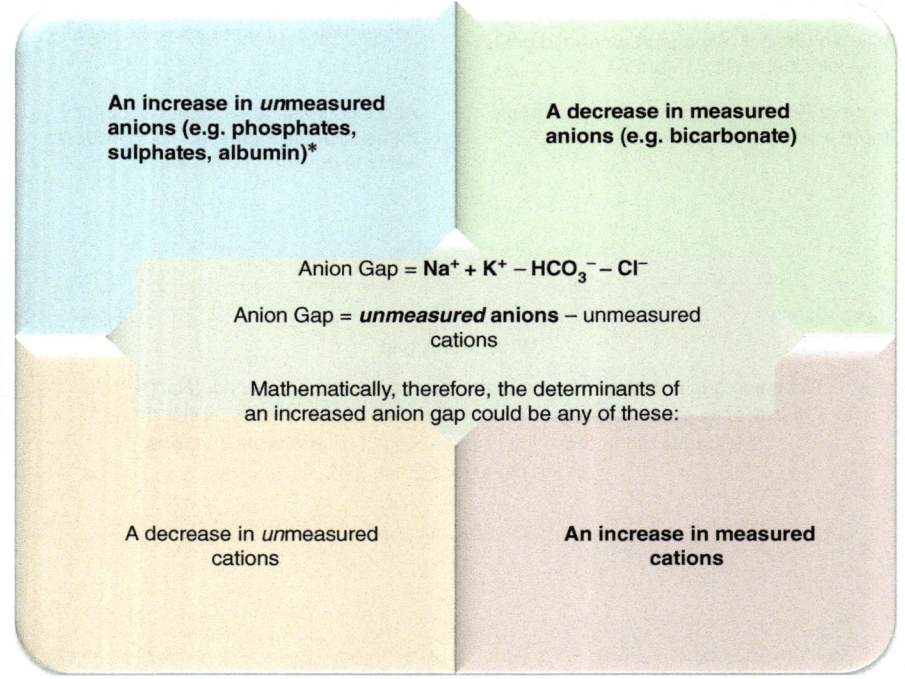

Gabow PA. Disorders associated with an altered anion gap. Kidney Int. 1985;27:472.

Rose BD, Post TW. Clinical physiology of acid-base and electrolyte disorders. 5th ed. New York: McGraw-Hill; 2001. p. 583–8.

9.5   Electrolytes That Influence the Anion Gap

Dyselectrolytemias can widen or narrow the anion gap.

Anion gap

$$AG = ([Na^+]+[K^+]) - ([Cl^-]+[HCO_3^-])$$

Or as just discussed,

$$AG = [\text{unmeasured anions}] - [\text{unmeasured cations}]$$

Increase in anion gap (>20 mEq/L)		**Decrease in anion gap (<7 mEq/L)**	
Can be due to:		Can be due to:	
Fall in unmeasured cations	**Rise in unmeasured anions**	**Rise in unmeasured cations**	**Fall in unmeasured anions**
Hypo-calcemia	Hyper-albuminemia (e.g., due to volume contraction)	Hyper-kalemia*	Hypo-albuminemia (see Sect. 9.9)
Hypo-magnesemia	Increase in organic anions	Hyper-magnesemia	
		Lithium intoxication	
		Paraprotein-emias	

*If the usual formula (the one that doesn't incorporate K^+ is used), K^+ is in that sense an unmeasured cation

9

Gabow PA. Disorders associated with an altered anion gap. Kidney Int. 1985;27:472.

9.6   The Derivation of the Anion Gap

The Law of Electroneutrality can also be written as follows:

Total cations – total anions = 0

$$[Na^+] + [K^+] - [Cl^-] - [HCO_3^-] - [A^-] - [unmeasured\ anions] = 0$$

In the above equation,

[H⁺] is not taken into consideration since its concentration relative to other cations is miniscule.

The concentration of the **unmeasured anions** (e.g. PO_4^- and SO_4^-) is only to the order of 1–3 mEq/L (average 2 mEq/L).

The symbol **[A⁻]** signifies the collective base pairs of the other weak acids: mostly the charged amino acid residues of plasma proteins.

[A⁻]

These weak acids are 90 % dissociated at the body pH of 7.4 (since their pK ranges from 6.6 to 6.8). A_{tot} or the total concentration of these weak acids is 2.4 times (in mEq/L) the concentration of plasma proteins (in g/dL).

$$[A^-] = A_{tot} \times 0.9$$

$[A^-]$ = Plasma protein concentration in g/dL x 2.4 x 0.9

$[A^-]$ now becomes quantifiable, and based on the normal range of plasma proteins, its normal range is seen to be 11–16.

Substituting the normal values of the ions in the equation

$$[Na^+] + [K^+] - [Cl^-] - [HCO_3^-] - [A^-] - [unmeasured\ anions] = 0$$

We have:

$$140 + 4 - 102 - 25 - 15 - 2 = 0$$

The normal range for the anion gap is 10–15.

9

Smith RM. Evaluation of arterial blood gases and acid-base homeostasis. In: Manual of clinical problems in pulmonary medicine. 6th ed. Philadelphia: Lippincott Williams and Wilkins; 2005.

9.7 Calculation of the Anion Gap

For the calculation of anion gap either of the two following formulae can be used:

$[Na^+] - [Cl^-] - [HCO_3^-]$	$[Na^+] + [K^+] - [Cl^-] - [HCO_3^-]$
Normal range: 12±4 mEq/L	*Normal range: 16±mEq/L*
This is the generally used formula. K^+ is excluded from the formula on the grounds that the value of K^+ is generally small enough to be disregarded.	This is the formula used when the value of K^+ is expected to vary significantly, as in renal patients.

Newer autoanalysers report the normal serum Cl^- at a higher value (than did the "older" machines); the normal range for the anion gap with the newer machines is lower, usually ranging between 3 and 11 mEq/L. However, given that its measurement hinges on multiple factors, a wide AG can be diagnosed with assurance when above 17–18 mEq/L.

Either venous CO_2 or the arterial HCO_3^- can be used in the formula:	
$AG = [Na^+] - [Cl^-] - venous\ CO_2$	$AG = [Na^+] - [Cl^-] - [HCO_3^-]$
As far as possible the venous CO_2 should be used in the calculation; this is the preferred approach.	Venous CO_2 roughly approximates the calculated arterial HCO_3^-, so the latter is often used in its place.

9

Goodkin DA, Krishna GG, Narins RG. The role of anion gap in detecting and managing mixed metabolic acid–base disorders. Clin Endocrinol Metabol. 1984;13:333–49.

Martin L. All you really need to know to interpret arterial blood gases. Philadelphia: Lippincott Williams and Wilkins; 1999.

Paulson WD, Gallah MF. Diagnosis of mixed acid-base disorders in diabetic ketoacidosis. Am J Med Sci. 1993;306:295–300.

Sadjadi SA. A new range for the anion gap. Ann Intern Med. 1995;123:807.

9.8   Causes of a Wide-Anion-Gap Metabolic Acidosis

Abnormal *endogenous* generation of anions	Lactic acidosis
	Type 1 (hypoperfusion)
	Type 2 (deranged carbohydrate metabolism)
	Ketoacidosis Diabetic ketoacidosis Alcoholic ketoacidosis Starvation ketoacidosis
	Renal acidosis Uremia Acute renal failure
Ingestion of *exogenous* toxin and drugs	Methanol Ethylene glycol Salicylate

It is not generally appreciated that metabolic alkalosis can sometimes cause a widening of the anion gap.

Causes of a wide anion gap in metabolic *alkalosis*		
Contraction of extracellular volume can increase the concentration of plasma albumin	Increase in the net negative charges on the surface of the albumin molecules	Increase in lactate production in response to the alkalosis
The magnitude of this widening is generally small.		

9

Emmett M. Anion-gap interpretation: the old and the new. Nat Clin Prac. 2006;2:4.

Gabow PA. Disorders associated with an altered anion gap. Kidney Int. 1985;27:472.

Madias NE, Ayus JC, Adrogue HJ. Increased anion gap in metabolic alkalosis: the role of plasma-protein equivalency. N Engl J Med. 1979;300:1421.

9.9   The Corrected Anion Gap (AG$_c$)

Certain factors can limit the diagnostic accuracy of the AG:

Errors of measurement	Since the measurement of three to four ions is required in its computation, there are greater chances of errors in its measurement.
Lactic acidosis	In lactic acidosis the AG may sometimes remain normal in spite of the presence of a significant acidosis.
Hypo-albumin-emia	The albumin molecule carries a large number of negative charges on its surface; therefore albumin accounts for most of the unmeasured anions. Albumin is normally responsible for virtually all of the value of the AG. *'Low Albumin, Low Anion gap'*: For every gram per dL decrease in albumin below 4.4 g/dL, the AG narrows by 2.5–3 mmol/L. The anion gap can be spuriously low when significant hypoalbuminemia exists. In severe hypoalbuminemia (such as in the nephrotic syndrome and cirrosis), a wide anion gap metabolic acidosis may exist, masked by hypoalbuminemia.

Corrected Anion Gap (AG$_c$)

The AG$_c$ is an anion gap adjusted for the albumin and phosphate:

$$AG_c = ([Na^+ + K^+] - [Cl^- + HCO_3^-]) - (2\,[\text{Albumin in g/dL}]) + 0.5\,[\text{Phosphate in mg/dL}] - \text{Lactate}$$

or,

$$AG_c = ([Na^+ + K^+] - [Cl^- + HCO_3^-]) - (2\,[\text{Albumin in g/dL}]) + 1.5\,[\text{Phosphate in mmol/L}] - \text{Lactate}$$

9

Feldman M, Soni N, Dickson B. Influence of hypoalbuminemia or hyperalbuminemia on the serum anion gap. J Lab Clin Med. 2005;146:317.

Figge J, Jabor A, Kazda A. Anion gap and hypoalbuminemia. Crit Care Med. 1998;26 (11):1807–10.

Gabow PA. Disorders associated with an altered anion gap. Kidney Int. 1985;27:472.

De Troyer A, Stolarczyk A, Zegersdebeyl D, Stryckmans P. Value of anion-gap determination in multiple myeloma. N Engl J Med. 1977;296:858–860.

9.10   Clues to the Presence of Metabolic Acidosis

The anion gap provides important diagnostic clues to the presence of certain underlying disorders.

HCO_3 or TCO_2 (see Sect. 9.19) is low	Serum chloride is elevated	Anion gap is high

Firstly, a wide anion gap indicates the presence of a metabolic acidosis. As a rule of the thumb, *when AG > 30 mMol/L metabolic acidosis is almost invariably present*. When AG 20–29 mMol/L, metabolic acidosis is present in two-thirds of the time.* Secondly, since the AG is wide in some etiologies of metabolic acidosis and not in others, a *wide* AG helps narrow down the differential diagnosis by eliminating the causes of a *normal* anion gap metabolic acidosis (NAGMA).

*Lactic acidosis, diabetic ketoacidosis and alcoholic ketoacidosis can result in a substantially raised anion gap. It is unusual for the anion gap to be widened more than about 20 mEq/L in starvation ketoacidosis.

Gabow PA, Kaehny WD, Fennessy PV, et al. Diagnostic importance of an increased serum anion gap. N Engl J Med. 1980;303:854.

Oster JR, Perez GO, Materson BJ. Use of the anion gap in clinical medicine. South Med J. 1988;81:229.

Rose BD, Post TW. Clinical physiology of acid-base and electrolyte disorders. 5th ed. New York: McGraw-Hill; 2001. p. 583–8.

9.11   Normal Anion-Gap Metabolic Acidosis

Lost bicarbonate is replaced by chloride; as a result the anion gap remains unaltered, i.e., it remains within normal limits. Because there is a rise in serum chloride, normal anion gap metabolic acidosis is also referred to as hyperchloremic acidosis.

Loss of bicarbonate or its precursors			Retention of acids
Loss of bicarbonate precursors	**Renal loss of bicarbonate**	**Gastrointestinal loss of bicarbonate**	**Decreased renal excretion of fixed acids**
Recovery phase of diabetic ketoacidosis	*The kidney conserves Na⁺ in an attempt to protect the fluid volume; the Na⁺ is retained as NaCl; this results in a net gain of chloride*	*The kidney conserves Na⁺ in an attempt to protect the fluid volume; again, the Na⁺ is retained as NaCl, resulting in a net gain of chloride*	-Type 1 RTA
	-Type 2 RTA	-Diarrhea	-Type 4 RTA
	-Carbonic inhibitor use	-Loss or drainage of pancreatic secretions	-Chronic renal failure
		-Uretero-sigmoidostomy	
		-Small bowel fistula	

See also Sects. 9.11 and 9.12

9

Rose BD, Post TW. Clinical physiology of acid-base and electrolyte disorders. 5th ed. New York: McGraw-Hill; 2001. p. 583–8.

Winter SD, Pearson JR, Gabow PA, et al. The fall of the serum anion gap. Arch Intern Med. 1990;150:311.

9.12 Pathogenesis of Normal-Anion Gap Metabolic Acidosis

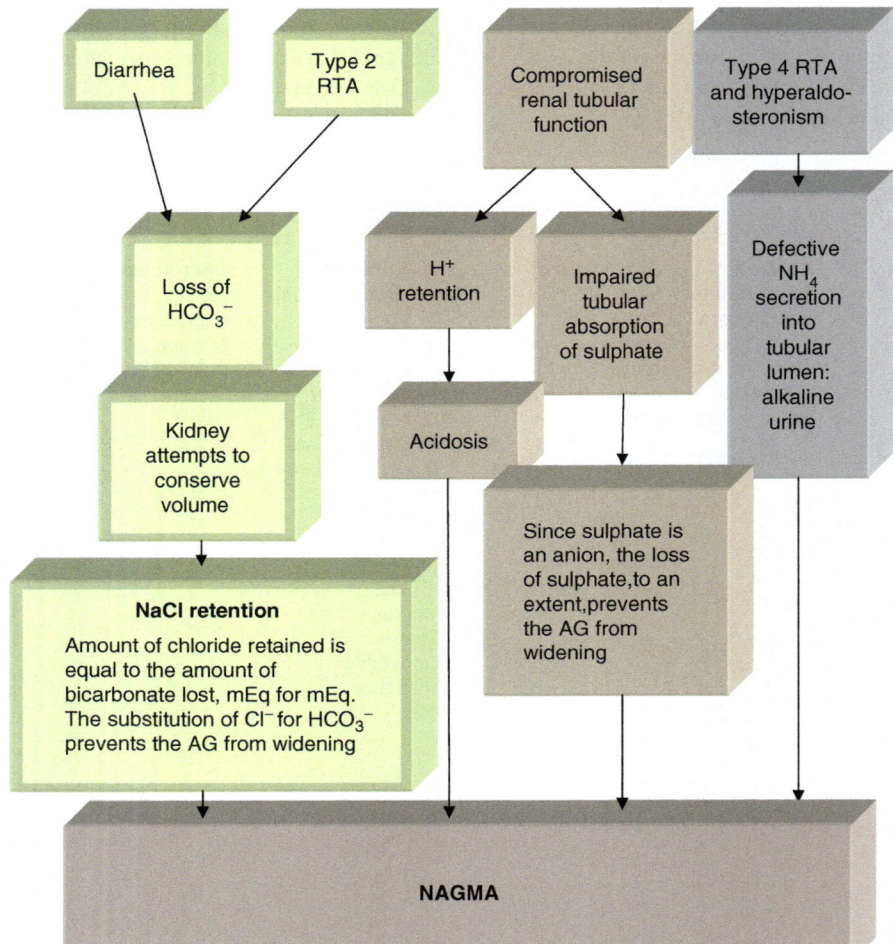

9.13   Negative Anion Gap

Rarely the anion gap may have a negative value: if the sum of the measured anions exceeds the sum of the measured cations.

Looking at the following equation, it is possible to understand why each of the above derangements can result in a **low or negative anion gap**:

$$\text{Anion gap} = [Na^+] - [Cl^-] - [HCO_3^-]$$

Underestimation of serum sodium	Overestimation of serum chloride	High serum bromide levels
In severe *hypernatremia* the Na⁺ concentration may be underestimated and may actually be much higher than the measured Na⁺ concentration.	In severe *hyperlipidemia* the caloric method grossly overestimates the serum chloride.	Chronic pyridostigmine bromide therapy for myasthenia gravis results in high serum bromide levels. Most laboratories report the bromide as chloride.
Hyponatremia	**Hyperchloremia**	**'Pseudohyperchloremia'**

9

Faradji-Hazan V, Oster JR, Fedeman DG, et al. Effect of pyridostigmine bromide on serum bicarbonate concentration and the anion gap. J Am Soc Nephrol. 1991;1:1123.

Graber ML, Quigg RJ, Stempsey WE, Weis S. Spurious hyperchloremia and decreased anion gap in hyperlipidemia. Ann Intern Med. 1983;98:607.

Kelleher SP, Raciti A, Arbeit LA. Reduced or absent serum anion gap as a marker for severe lithium carbonate intoxication. Arch Intern Med. 1986;146:1839.

9.14   Systemic Consequences of Metabolic Acidosis

Circulatory effects of metabolic acidosis		
Direct effect of the acidosis on arteries	**Effects of catecholamine release** Acidemia (unless severe) will' by activating the sympathetic nervous system (and increasing catecholamine levels), often offset its own direct effects on the circulation.	
Arteriodilation (Acidemia can directly dilate the peripheral arterioles).	*Arterioconstriction* • Tachycardia • Arrythmias	*Venoconstriction* The increased venous return results in pulmonary congestion, elevated PA pressures and pulmonary edema.

Cardiac effects of metabolic acidosis		
Severe metabolic acidosis	**Mild to moderate metabolic acidosis:** *Either of the following are possible:*	
Myocardial depression (Acidemia directly depresses cardiac function when severe).	*Direct myocardial depression* There is impairment in cardiac contractility, and a reduced response to circulating catecholamines.	*Myocardial stimulation* Catecholamine release occurs as a consequence of the acidosis. There is a lowered threshold for arrythmias.

Severe acidemia can actually blunt the sympathetic activation that is present at milder levels, and the ensuing arteriodilatation and myocardial depression can result in cardiovascular collapse. Severe acidemia can also predispose to arrythmias.

9

Gonzalez NC, Clancy RL. Inotropic and intracellular acid-base changes during metabolic acidosis. Am J Physiol. 1975;228:1060–4.

Marsh JD, Margolis TI, Kim D. Mechanism of diminished contractile response to catecholamines during acidosis. Am J Physiol. 1988;254:H20–7.

Mitchell JH, Wildenthal K, Johnson RL Jr. The effects of acid-base disturbance on cardiovascular and pulmonary function. Kidney Int. 1972;1:375–89.

Orchard CH, Cingolani HE. Acidosis and arrhythmias in cardiac muscle. Cardiovasc Res. 1994;28:1312–9.

Orchard CH, Kentish JC. Effects of changes of pH on the contractile function of cardiac muscle. Am J Physiol. 1990;258:C967.

Shapiro JI. Functional and metabolic responses of isolated hearts to acidosis: effect of sodium bicarbonate and Carbicarb. Am J Physiol. 1990;258:H1835.

9.15   Other Systemic Consequences of Metabolic Acidosis

Respiratory	Hyper-ventilation, dyspnea (metabolic acidosis stimulates ventilation).
	Increased pulmonary vascular resistance: pulmonary edema.
	Reduced diaphragmatic strength: respiratory muscle fatigue.
	Acute acidosis results in increased oxygen delivery to tissues; in chronic acidosis, in contrast, oxygen delivery to the tissues decreases.
Metabolic	Insulin resistance
Cerebral	Dysregulated metabolism and regulation of cell volume: altered sensorium, drowsiness presumably due to an osmotic disequilibrium between the brain cells and the CSF.
Renal	Renal hypertrophy (promotes acid excretion and thereby helps restore acid-base imbalance; however may be detrimental when renal insufficiency exists.
	Nephrocalcinosis and nephrolithiasis (reduced citrate excretion helps the body conserve its alkali, but also reduces the solubility of calcium in the urine).
	Possible complement-related and oxidant-related renal damage
Bone	Decalcification: by promoting parathormone release
Muscle	Catabolism

9

Alpern RJ. Trade-offs in the adaptation to acidosis. Kidney Int. 1995;47:1205–15.

Bailey JL, Mitch WE. Metabolic acidosis as a uremic toxin. Semin Nephrol. 1996;16:160–6.

Bergofsky EH, Lehr DE, Fishman AP. The effect of changes in hydrogen ion concentration on the pulmonary circulation. J Clin Invest. 1962;41:1492–502.

Bushinsky DA. Stimulated osteoclastic and suppressed osteoblastic activity in metabolic but not respiratory acidosis. Am J Physiol. 1995;268:C80–8.

Bushinsky DA. The contribution of acidosis to renal osteodystrophy. Kidney Int. 1995;47:1816–32.

Bushinsky DA, Sessler NE. Critical role of bicarbonate in calcium release from bone. Am J Physiol. 1992;263:F510–5.

Garibotto G, Russo R, Sofia A, et al. Skeletal muscle protein synthesis and degradation in patients with chronic renal failure. Kidney Int. 1994;45:1432–9.

Guisado R, Arieff AI. Neurologic manifestations of diabetic comas: correlation with biochemical alterations in the brain. Metabolism. 1975;24:665–79.

9

Hamm LL. Renal handling of citrate. Kidney Int. 1990;38:728–35.

Hostetter TH. Progression of renal disease and renal hypertrophy. Annu Rev Physiol. 1995;57: 263–78.

Lemann J Jr., Bushinsky DA, Hamm LL. Bone buffering of acid and base in humans. Am J Physiol Renal Physiol. 2003;285:F811–32.

May RC, Kelly RA, Mitch WE. Metabolic acidosis stimulates protein degradation in rat muscle by a glucocorticoid- dependent mechanism. J Clin Invest. 1986;77:614–21.

Mitchell JH, Wildenthal K, Johnson RL Jr. The effects of acid-base disturbance on cardiovascular and pulmonary function. Kidney Int. 1972;1:375–89.

Wasserman K. Coupling of external to cellular respiration during exercise: the wisdom of the body revisited. Am J Physiol. 1994;266:E519–39.

Winegrad AI, Kern EFO, Simmons DA. Cerebral edema in diabetic ketoacidosis. N Engl J Med. 1985;312:1184–5.

9.16   Hyperkalemia and Hypokalemia in Metabolic Acidosis

Acidosis can result in hyperkalemia; conversely hyperkalemia can result in acidosis. For every 0.1 unit fall in extracellular pH, a rise of plasma K^+ by 0.2–1.7 mEq/L (average 0.6 mEq/L) can be anticipated. For a variety of reasons, the potassium levels in diabetic acidosis (DKA) can vary widely (see below), and K^+ levels must be closely monitored. For ill understood reasons, the magnitude of the hyperkalemia per unit fall in pH is somewhat less in DKA and lactic acidosis.

Mechanisms underlying hyperkalemia in metabolic acidosis:		Mechanisms underlying hypokalemia in Diabetic ketoacidosis (DKA).
Renal tubular conservation of H^+ in uremia.	H^+ enters cells, and K^+ shifts out of the intra-cellular compartment to maintain electroneutrality.	1. *Osmotic diuresis* 2. *Treatment of DKA by fluids:* • Hemodilution • Correction of metabolic acidosis 3. *Treatment of DKA by insulin therapy:* K^+ shifts back into the intracellular compartment.
Hyperkalemia or normokalemia can occur in spite of depleted body K^+ stores, but the K^+ will fall as the acidosis is corrected.		

Hyperkalemia can result in acidosis.

The entry of K^+ into cells is balanced by the efflux of H^+ out of the intracellular compartment to maintain electroneutrality.

In states of hyperkalemia such as *hyperaldosteronism*, the following events occur within the renal tubular cells:

Increased intracellular K^+ levels → Migration of H^+ out of the intracellular compartment* → Intracellular alkalosis → Decreased generation of ammonium → Decreased excretion of H^+

9

*In order to maintain electroneutrality

Adrogué HJ, Madias NE. Changes in plasma potassium concentration during acute acid-base disturbances. Am J Med. 1981;71:456.

Altenberg GA, Aristimuño PC, Amorena CE, Taquini AC. Amiloride prevents the metabolic acidosis of a KCl load in nephrectomized rats. Clin Sci (Lond). 1989;76:649.

Szylman P, Better OS, Chaimowitz C, Rosler A. Role of hyperkalemia in the metabolic acidosis of isolated hypoaldosteronism. N Engl J Med. 1976;294:361.

Wallia R, Greenberg AS, Piraino B, et al. Serum electrolyte patterns in end-stage renal disease. Am J Kidney Dis. 1986;8:98.

Wiederseiner JM, Muser J, Lutz T, et al. Acute metabolic acidosis: characterization and diagnosis of the disorder and the plasma potassium response. J Am Soc Nephrol. 2004;15:1589.

9.17   Compensatory Response to Metabolic Acidosis

Rarely does a metabolic acidosis remain uncompensated (examples: presence of associated respiratory disease; a paralysed patient on ventilator who is being given inappropriately low minute volumes). In contrast to respiratory disorders (which are well compensated by the kidney), compensation for metabolic disorders is rarely as perfect.

The lungs being much the quicker to respond, respiratory compensation for metabolic disorders begins faster than does the renal compensation for respiratory disorders.

Metabolic Compensation		Respiratory compensation
When the kidney is not the primary cause for the metabolic acidosis, it will help in the compensatory processes.		Hyperventilation occurs as a result of stimulation of central and peripheral chemo-receptors.
Hydrogen ions combine with NH_3 to form NH_4. There is increased synthesis of NH_3 (from glutamine) in the face of an acid load. $NH_3+H^+ \rightarrow NH_4$. NH_4 is excreted in the urine (see Sect.4.3) This is the principal renal compensatory mechanism.	**Hydrogen ions combine with HPO_4^- to form $H_2PO_4^-$** $H_2PO_4^-$ is excreted in the urine.	Hyperventilation is a rapid response that starts within minutes. *A fall of $PaCO_2$ by 1.2 mmHg occurs for every 1 mEq/L fall in HCO_3.* Metabolic acidosis can become life threatening if the lungs are prevented from responding in this manner to the acidosis (such as when inappropriately low minute volumes are dispensed on a controlled mode of mechanical ventilation.

9

9.18 Compensation for Metabolic Acidosis

Winter's formula	ΔPCO_2	PCO_2 and pH
The degree of compensation can be predicted by Winter's formula: *Predicted PCO_2 = $(1.5 \times HCO_3^-) + 8 +/- 2$.* **Lower PCO_2** values than predicted indicate the presence of a coexisting respiratory alkalosis. **Higher CO_2** values than predicted indicate a coexisting respiratory acidosis.	The change in PCO_2 (ΔPCO_2) = $(1.1-1.3) \times \Delta HCO_3$	*Predicted PCO_2 = the last 2 digits of the pH*

Limits of compensation for metabolic acidosis

- Although respiratory response to metabolic acidosis starts immediately, the overall compensatory response takees 12–24 h to develop fully.

- The lungs are capable of maximising ventilation such that the PCO_2 drops to a lower limit of about 10 mmHg.

9

Smith RM. Evaluation of arterial blood gases and acid-base homeostasis. In: Manual of clinical problems in pulmonary medicine. 6th ed. Philadelphia: Lippincott Williams and Wilkins; 2005.

9.19   Total CO$_2$ (TCO$_2$)

TCO$_2$ is the sum of all the species that can potentially generate CO$_2$.

Bicarbonate (HCO$_3^-$)			
HCO$_3^-$ is the only one of the CO$_2^-$ producing species that is present in the body in significant amounts. TCO$_2$ usually corresponds to the **venous** bicarbonate level, which itself parallels the **arterial** bicarbonate. Therefore the arterial HCO$_3^-$ can be guessed at with reasonable accuracy from the TCO$_2$ without having to resort to arterial puncture.	H$_2$CO$_3$	Carb-amino CO$_2$	Dissolved CO$_2$
	The concentration of these three species is generally insignificant and can be disregarded.		

Most of the contribution to TCO$_2$ comes from the bicarbonate. A relatively miniscule contribution comes from dissolved CO$_2$.

Acute respiratory disturbances	Chronic respiratory disturbances	Metabolic disturbances
In acute respiratory disturbances, the bicarbonate remains relatively unchanged.	Chronic respiratory disturbances do result in a significant alteration in bicarbonate levels as a result of renal compensatory processes.	It is the metabolic disturbances that primarily alter the bicarbonate.
Acute respiratory disturbances produce only minor changes in TCO$_2$.	Chronic respiratory disturbances produce appreciable changes in TCO$_2$.	Metabolic disturbances produce the greatest changes in TCO$_2$.

9

9.20   Altered Bicarbonate Is Not Specific for a Metabolic Derangement

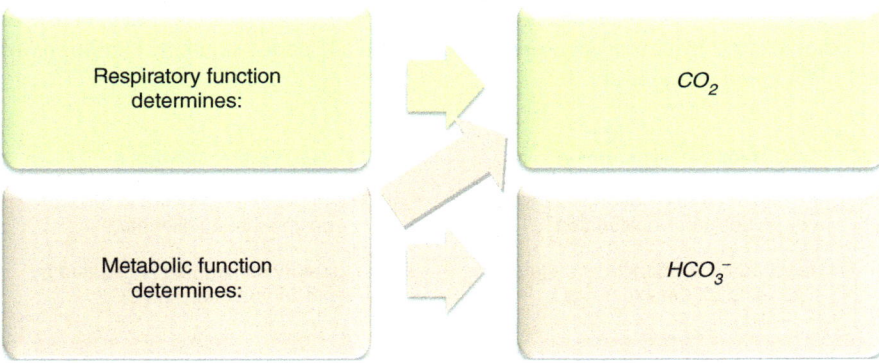

Although plasma bicarbonate is the most commonly used index of the *metabolic* status, it can also be altered in *respiratory* disturbances.

Since HCO_3^- is determined by both metabolic and repiratory phenomena, an alered HCO_3^- does not reflect an exclusive metabolic process. To negate the effect of respiratory disturbances on the diagnostic utility of HCO_3^-, two other indices are employed (see following section):

Standard bicarbonate   **Base exess**

9

9.21   Actual Bicarbonate and Standard Bicarbonate

Standard bicarbonate (SBC) is the concentration of HCO_3^- in the plasma of blood that has been fully oxygenated and equilibriated with a PCO_2 of 40 mmHg at 37 °C. In other words, SBC is a measure of plasma HCO_3 under standard conditions of PO_2, PCO_2 and temperature.

Respiratory acidosis	Respiratory alkalosis
Plasma sample from a patient in respiratory acidosis is equilibriated	Plasma sample from a patient in respiratory acidosis is equilibriated
The respiratory component is negated by blowing off the excess CO_2.	The respiratory component is negated by replacing the deficient CO_2.

The sample is analysed for HCO_3 when CO_2 has been restored to 40 mmHg.

The bicarbonate in the sample now should reflect the metabolic component only. This "adjusted" bicarbonate is called the *standard bicarbonate*.

In health the actual bicarbonate equals the standard bicarbonate.

Note, that with standard blood gas analyzers, only the respiratory parameters (i.e. PCO_2 and PO_2) can be *directly measured*. The values of the metabolic parameters, i.e. plasma bicarbonate, standard bicarbonate, base excess (Sect. 9.20) and whole blood buffer base (Sect. 9.23) are all *derived*.

9

9.22 Relationship Between ABC and SBC

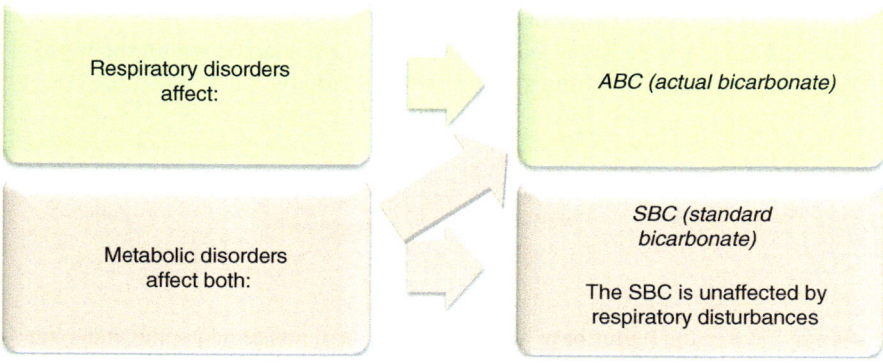

Standard bicarbonate is therefore more specific for metabolic disturbances. The relationship between ABC and SBC indicates the nature of the underlying disorder:

Metabolic disordrs				Respiratory disoders		
In metabolic disorders, both ABC and SBC are altered in the same directions.				In respiratory disorders, ABC and SBC are altered in different direction.		
Pure metabolic acidosis		Pure metabolic alkalosis		ABC > SBC	ABC = SBC	ABC < SBC
				Respiratory alkalosis	No respiratory disturbance	Respiratory acidosis
ABC low	SBC low	ABC high	SBC high			

9

9.23 Buffer Base

Syn: Whole buffer base (Singer and Hastings, 1948).

The buffer base is the sum of all the base anions contained within the blood. It includes the important buffering systems within the body:

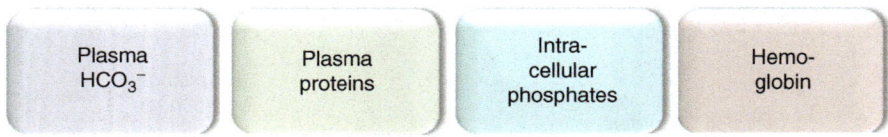

It may be that the buffer base mirrors electrolyte derangements, the understanding of which may hold the key to this elusive concept. In respiratory disturbances the buffer base reserve is preserved.

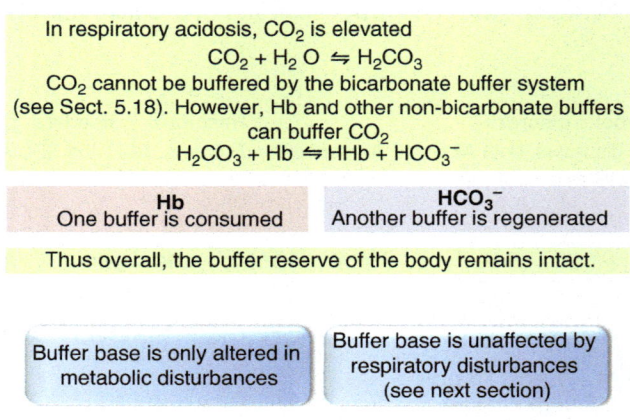

Hopley L, van Schalkwyk J, editors. "Bluffer base". In: Acid-base balance: common ground? www.anaesthetist.com. Last updated: 24 Sept 2006. Last accessed 13 May 2012.

9.24 Base Excess

In 1958, Astrup and Siggard-Andersen described *Base Excess* (BE) as an improved indicator of *metabolic* acid–base disorders.

Under standard conditions (PCO_2 of 40 mmHg at 37 °C):

"Positive" base excess:	**"Negative" base excess:**
Metabolic alkalosis	*Metabolic acidosis*
The amount of acid that needs to be added to return the pH of 1 liter of an alkalemic blood sample to 7.40.	The amount of alkali that needs to be added to return the pH of 1 liter of an acidic blood sample to 7.40.

Standard base excess
Calculated as for blood with a haemoglobin concentration of 5 g/dL (5 g/dL reflects the buffering capacity of hemoglobin averaged out for the whole body including the extracellular fluid).

Base excess is expressed in mEq/L, and is normally zero (range: +2 to −2). Because of its lower SpO_2, the BE of venous blood (unless oxygenated) is higher than that of arterial blood (2–2.5 mEq/L).

For a normal Hb concentration, the following relationship holds between BE and *changes in SBC* (ΔSBC):

$$BE = 1.3 \times \Delta SBC$$

Both SBC and Base Excess (Sect. 9.20) were originally conceived as parameters that would purely reflect metabolic events to the exclusion of respiratory events. This does not apply in vivo, since any changes in PCO_2 induce corresponding changes in non-bicarbonate buffers.

9

Barry A. Utility of standard base excess in acid base analysis (editorial). Crit Care Med. 1998;26(7):1146–7.

Gennari FJ, Cohen JJ, Kassirer JP. Measurement of acid-base status. In: Cohen JJ, Kassirer JP, editors. Acid/base. Boston: Little, Brown; 1982.

Schlichtig R, Grogono AW, Severinghaus JW. Human $PaCO_2$ and standard base excess compensation for acid-base imbalance. Crit Care Med. 1998;28:1173–9.

9.25   Ketosis and Ketoacidosis

Diabetic ketoacidosis	Diagnosed by the suggestive triad of **hyperglycemia** (plasma glucose >250 mg/dL), **ketonemia** (after 1:1 dilution, serum ketones "large positive" by the semi-quantitative nitroprusside test) and **acidosis**, in the presence of compatible symptoms. This triad is however *neither sensitive* (e.g., a counterbalancing disorder may negate the acidosis); *nor specific* (see below). Betahydroxy butyric acid (the dominant ketone excreted in urine) is not measurable by the usual semi-quantitative methods. Although typically the anion gap is widened early on (WAGMA), sizeable ketone losses can prevent a significant widening of the anion gap. Later during the course of its therapy, a NAGMA is the usual form of acidosis in DKA (Sect.9.27).
Starvation ketosis	In prolonged fasting, decreased insulin levels result in the breakdown of adipocytes into free fatty acids. Fats become the fuel for most tissues (sparing glucose for oxidation by the brain) and may comprise up to 80 % of energy expenditure; this leads to ketosis: up to 1,500 mmol of ketoacids may be produced each day. After several weeks of fasting, the acidosis is fully developed, but preserved insulin secretion (though decreased) is adequate to prevent hyperglycemia and gross ketosis. The acidemia is consequently mild (pH > 7.3; HCO_3^- >17 mEq/L) and responds well to glucose administration. Ketonuria is typically heavy in contrast to the relatively slight ketonemia.
Alcoholic ketosis	The acid-base disorder may be complicated by the associated respiratory alkalosis of chronic liver disease, the metabolic alkalosis of vomiting and the metabolic (lactic) acidosis of pancreatitis. This leads to a variable pH. The ratio of serum betahydroxybutyric acid to acetoacetate in much higher than in DKA (in all ketotic states this ratio is at least 2:1 or 3:1). In contrast to starvation ketosis, the acidemia may be more severe. The osmolar gap is frequently widened (on account of acetone and ethanol itself) and serum uric acid levels may be high (ketoacids compete with uric acid for tubular excretion).

9

Gennari JF, Adrogue HJ, Galla JH, Madias NE. Acid base disorders and their treatment. Boca Raton: Taylor and Francis; 2005. p. 228–9.

Kamel KS, Lin SH, Cheema-Dhadli S, Marliss EB, Halperin ML. Prolonged total fasting: a feast for the integrative physiologist. Kidney Int. 1998;53:531–9.

Oster JR, Epstein M. Acid-base aspects of ketoacidosis. Am J Nephrol. 1984;4:137–51.

9.26   Acidosis in Untreated Diabetic Ketoacidosis

Diabetic ketoacidosis
Ketoacids are produced mainly in the hepatocytes. One H^+ ion is generated from the dissociation of each keto-ion (e.g., beta-hydroxy butyric acid, acetoacetic acid).

Acidosis:	**Widened anion gap:** The H^+ is buffered, consuming HCO_3 and widening the anion gap.

High anion gap metabolic acidosis
However other acid-base disorders can enter into the equation:

Dehydration and circulatory failure.	Vomiting: loss of the chloride-rich acidic gastric secretions.
Lactic acidosis	**Metabolic alkalosis**
Increased co-production of NAD$^+$ with lactate More beta-hydroxy butyric acid is produced relative to acetoacetic acid.	
Lactic acidosis can mask ketosis Since the usual nitroprusside test for ketones involves the testing of acetoacetic acid (rather than beta-hydroxy butyric acid), this test may be falsely negative.	

9

Adrogué HJ, Wilson H, Boyd AE III, et al. Plasma acid-base patterns in diabetic ketoacidosis. N Engl J Med. 1982;307:1603.

Rose BD, Post TW. Clinical physiology of acid-base and electrolyte disorders. 5th ed. New York: McGraw-Hill. 2001. p. 583–8.

9.27   Acidosis in Diabetic Ketoacidosis Under Treatment

Treatment of DKA can convert a high anion gap metabolic acidosis into a normal anion gap metabolic acidosis.

Volume expansion and increased renal excretion of ketones
Ketones (anions) are excreted through the kidneys as salts of sodium and potassium (cations).

Acidosis	**Narrow anion gap**
Since ketones are precursors of bicarbonate, the loss of ketones, is effectively, loss of bicarbonate.	However, the lost bicarbonate is replaced by chloride from:
The loss of bicarbonate would normally be expected to result in a *wide anion gap.*	• Saline resuscitation • Gastrointestinal absorption • Renal absorption *This narrows the anion gap*

Normal anion gap metabolic acidosis
In fact, *both* wide and normal anion gap metabolic acidosis may be present even before treatment is commenced; a clue to the existence of the latter may be found in the delta ratio (Sect. 9.36).

9

Oh MS, Carroll HJ, Goldstein DA, Fein IA. Hyperchloremic acidosis during the recovery phase of diabetic ketosis. Ann Intern Med. 1978;89:925.

9.28   Renal Mechanisms of Acidosis

The anatomic site of the pathology determines the type of acidosis that develops.

| WAGMA: Results mostly from glomerular pathology | NAGMA: Results mostly from renal tubular pathology |

Decrease in GFR

Since glomerular function is deranged, *the increase in H+ is proportional to the decrease in GFR.*

Glomerular function is mostly preserved; *the increase in H+ is out of proportion to the decrease in GFR*.* An increased tubular excretion of sulphate (as Na^+ or K^+) keeps the anion gap normal.

Hyper-chloremia

Chloride ions replace the lost bicarbonate: this also has a moderating effect on the anion gap.

Acidosis

Impaired excretion of fixed acids

Wide anion gap

Impaired excretion of anions (SO_4^-, urates).

Wide anion gap metabolic acidosis

Normal anion gap metabolic acidosis

*On occasion, in chronic renal failure, tubular function may be affected.

9

Rose BD, Post TW. Clinical physiology of acid-base and electrolyte disorders. 5th ed. New York: McGraw-Hill; 2001. p. 583–8.

Wallia R, Greenberg AS, Piraino B, et al. Serum electrolyte patterns in end-stage renal disease. Am J Kidney Dis. 1986;8:98.

9.29   L-Lactic Acidosis and D-Lactic Acidosis

Lactic acidosis is probably the commonest cause of metabolic acidosis in the hospitalized patient: tissue hypoxia is the usual cause. To define the disorder, the serum lactate should be at least 5 mEq/L (with associated metabolic acidosis).

> About 1 mEq/kg/h lactate is normally produced during glucose metabolism; it is utilized for gluconeogenesis by the liver.
>
> Normal serum lactate is generally ≤ 2 mEq/L. This can rise to about 4 mEq/L during exercise.

L-lactic acidosis		D-Lactic acidosis
Type A lactic acidosis occurs in states of tissue hypoperfusion Circulatory failure and shock Severe anemia Histotoxic hypoxia (CO or cyanide poisoning) Mitochondrial enzyme defects	**Type B (aerobic)** **B1**: *Underlying disease* (e.g., ketoacidosis, hepatic and renal failure, malignancy, leukaemia, lymphoma, infections (malaria, cholera, AIDS). **B2**: *Drugs and toxins* (e.g., biguanides, methanol, ethanol, cyanide, β-agonists, nitroprusside, INH, anti-retroviral drugs). **B3**: *Associated with inborn errors of metabolism* (e.g., pyruvate dehydrogenase deficiency).	D-lactate overproduction occurs when unabsorbed carbohydrate reaches normal colonic bacteria*. *Occurs in the setting of:* Intestinal obstruction Jejunoileal bypass A D-lactic acidosis must be suspected in the setting of unexplained metabolic acidosis especially if diarrhea is also present. A test for D-lactic acid needs to be separately ordered.

*The mammalian liver lacks D-lactic acid dehydrogenase and will therefore not properly metabolize D-lactic acid.

Cohen R, Woods H. Clinical and biochemical aspects of lactic acidosis. Oxford: Blackwell Scientific Publications; 1976.

Halperin ML, Kamel KS. D-Lactic acidosis: turning sugars into acids in the gastrointestinal tract. Kidney Int. 1996;49:1–8.

Lalau JD, Lacroix C, Compagnon P, de Cagny B, Rigaud JP, et al. Role of metformin accumulation in metformin- associated lactic acidosis. Diabetes Care. 1995;18:779–84.

McKenzie R, Fried MW, Sallie R, et al. Hepatic failure and lactic acidosis due to fialuridine (FIAU), an investigational nucleoside analogue for chronic hepatitis B. N Engl J Med. 1995;333:1099–105.

Steiner D, Williams RH. Respiratory inhibition and hypoglycemia by biguanides and decamethylenediguanide. Biochim Biophys Acta. 1958;30:329.

Stolberg L, Rolfe R, Gitlin N, et al. D-Lactic acidosis due to abnormal gut flora. N Engl J Med. 1982;306:1344.

9.30 Diagnosis of Specific Etiologies of Wide Anion Gap Metabolic Acidosis

Lactic acidosis	Wide anion-gap metabolic acidosis (WAGMA) in the absence of ketosis and uremia; negative history of alcohol or toxin ingestion. *Associated hyperphosphatemia* (from extracellular migration of phosphates), *hyperuricemia* (tubular urate secretion is competitively inhibited by lactate). Usually, *normal serum potassium.* Blood or plasma lactate levels greater than 4–5 mmol/L. (Note: venous lactate concentrations are approximately 50–100 % higher compared to arterial lactate levels). D-Lactate assays in the appropriate setting (see Sect. 9.29)
Methanol, ethylene glycol or paraldehyde.	WAGMA without ketosis or uremia; there may be a history of substance abuse. (Note: the wide anion gap can result as much from increased lactic acid levels as with abnormal anionic metabolites). Methanol: blood methanol (measured using gas chromatography in special labs; results may take severel days), serum formate (a better test later in the course of the illness), urine for myoglobin. Ethylene glycol: blood levels, urine for calcium oxalate crystals.
Salicylate poisoning	WAGMA without ketosis or uremia; history of acute aspirin overdose or chronic consumption (WAGMA is possibly due to organic acids, but likely multifactorial; lactic acidosis is responsible for the late component of salicylate-induced metabolic acidosis. The primary respiratory alkalosis that salicylates produce can worsen the metabolic acidosis). Plasma salicylate levels (therapeutic range:10–20 mg/dL).
Thiamine deficiency	WAGMA with clinical features of beriberi. Thiamine deficiency can also occur in patients on total parenteral nutrition (without micronutrient supplementation). Erythrocyte transketolase activity, blood and urine thiamine levels.

9

Fligner CL, Jack R, Twiggs GA, Raisys VA. Hyperosmolality induced by propylene glycol. A complication of silver sulfadiazine therapy. J Am Med Assoc. 1985;253:1606–9.

Gabow PA, Anderson RJ, Potts DE, Schrier RW, Acid-base disturbances in the salicylate- intoxication adult. Arch Intern Med. 1978;138:1481–4.

Gabow PA, Clay K, Sullivan JB, Lepoff R. Organic acids in ethylene glycol intoxication. Ann Intern Med. 1986;105:16–20.

Keller U, Mall T, Walter M, Bertel O, Mihatsch JM, Ritz R. Phaeochromocytoma with lactic acidosis. Br Med J. 1978;2:606–7.

Kreisberg RA, Owen WC, Siegel AM. Ethanol- induced hyperlactic-acidemia: inhibition of lactate utilization. J Clin Invest. 1971;50:166–74.

9

Lacouture PG, Wason S, Abrams A, Lovejoy FH Jr. Acute isopropyl alcohol intoxication. Diagnosis and management. Am J Med. 1983;75:680–6.

Lalau JD, Lacroix C, Compagnon P, de Cagny B, Rigaud JP, et al. Role of metformin accumulation in metformin- associated lactic acidosis. Diabetes Care. 1995;18:779–84.

McKenzie R, Fried MW, Sallie R, et al. Hepatic failure and lactic acidosis due to fialuridine (FIAU), an investigational nucleoside analogue for chronic hepatitis B. N Engl J Med. 1995; 333:1099–105.

O'Connor LR, Klein KL, Bethune JE. Hyperphosphatemia in lactic acidosis. N Engl J Med. 1977;297:707–9.

Romanski SA, Mc Mahon MM. Metabolic acidosis and thiamine deficiency. Mayo Clin Proc. 1999;74:259–63.

Steiner D, Williams RH. Respiratory inhibition and hypoglycemia by biguanides and decamethyl-enediguanide. Biochim Biophys Acta. 1958;30:329.

Velez RJ, Myers B, Guber MS. Severe acute metabolic acidosis (acute beri-beri): an avoidable complication of total parenteral nutrition. JPEN J Parenter Enteral Nutr. 1985;9:216–9.

Yu T. Effect of sodium lactate infusion on urate clearance in man. Proc Soc Exp Biol Med. 1957;96:809.

9.31 Pitfalls in the Diagnosis of Lactic Acidosis

Lactic acidosis	
Increased lactate Unlike in DKA, an anion (lactate) replaces bicarbonate.	*Increased H^+ retention*
Widened anion gap	*Acidosis*

Wide anion gap metabolic acidosis

Lactic acidosis usually results in a significant widening of the anion gap: if the anion gap is >30, an additional lactic acidosis should be suspected even if another obvious cause for wide-anion metabolic acidosis (e.g., renal failure), is obvious.

On occasion, lactic acidosis may be present without significant widening of the anion gap.

The source of the blood sample obtained may also influence the serum lactate

Venous blood	**Arterial blood**	**Mixed venous blood sampled by a pulmonary artery catheter**
Represents local lactate production: may be elevated if a tourniquet has been applied; if so, will not reflect systemic lactate levels.	Reflects production of lactate as well the ability of the liver to clear the lactate from the circulation.	It is possible that mixed venous blood provides the most accurate status of the blood lactate.

9

Weil MH, Michaels S, Rackow EC. Comparison of blood lactate concentrations in central venous, pulmonary artery and arterial blood. Crit Care Med. 1987;15:489–90.

9.32   Renal Tubular Acidosis

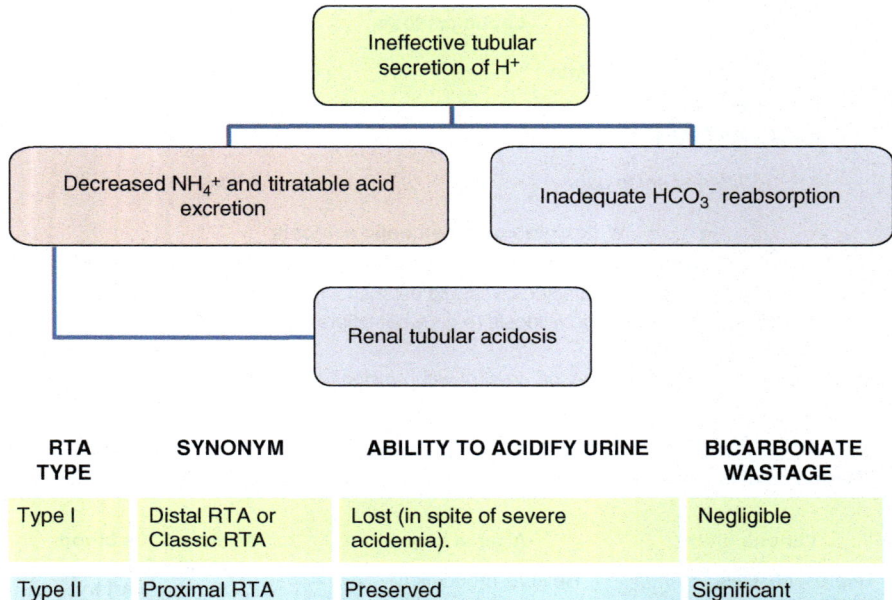

RTA TYPE	SYNONYM	ABILITY TO ACIDIFY URINE	BICARBONATE WASTAGE
Type I	Distal RTA or Classic RTA	Lost (in spite of severe acidemia).	Negligible
Type II	Proximal RTA with bicarbonate wastage RTA	Preserved	Significant
Type III	Distal RTA with bicarbonate wastage	Lost (despite severe acidemia).	Significant
Type IV	Hyperkalemic RTA associated with aldosterone deficiency	Preserved (in contrast to type I RTA).	None (in contrast to type II RTA).
Type V	Hyperkalemic distal RTA without aldosterone deficiency	Lost. A voltage-defect hinders both H^+ and K^+ secretion resulting in metabolic acidosis and hyperkalemia.	Negligible

9

Gennari FJ, Cohen JJ, Kassirer JP. Measurement of acid-base status. In: Cohen JJ, Kassirer JP, editors Acid/base. Boston: Little, Brown; 1982.

9.33   Distal RTA

Syn: Type I RTA, Classic RTA

A urinary acidifying defect results in a relatively alkaline urine (pH remains >5.5) in the face of severe acidemia. Distal RTA is generally more severe than proximal RTA.

Mechanisms:
- An ineffective proton pump
- A leaky tubular membrane that cannot prevent back-diffusion of H^+

Urinary bicarbonate loss		Renal wasting of sodium
		A high Na^+ load delivered to the distal tubule results in urinary loss of Na^+; this results in contraction of the ECF volume.
Systemic acidemia	Excretion of a high pH urine	**Secondary hyperaldosteronism**
Diagnostic test: The serum bicarbonate is made to fall (by acid loading) to about 15 mEq/L. If the urinary pH then remains >5.5, this is considered diagnostic of RTA.		Potassium loss in the urine

9

Caruana RJ, Buckalew VM Jr. The syndrome of distal (type 1) renal tubular acidosis. Medicine (Baltimore). 1988;67:84.

Rodriguez Soriano J. Renal tubular acidosis: the clinical entity. J Am Soc Nephrol. 2002;13:2160.

9.34   Mechanisms in Miscellaneous Causes of Normal Anion Gap Metabolic Acidosis

Catheter drainage of intestinal sectetions or enterocutaneous fistulas.	The secretions of both the small intestine (biliary, pancreatic) and large intestine are alkaline, and so loss of intestinal secretions results in alkalosis.
Secretory diarrhea Intestinal infections (e.g., viral infections, cholera), villous adenomas (see below) certain hormones (vasoactive intestinal peptide e.g., of neoplastic origin) and drugs.	All these can lead to HCO_3^- losses. The HCO_3^- that is lost is accompanied by Cl^-, and so the anion gap is preserved (NAGMA). In more severe cases, a WAGMA results when severe contraction of ECF leads to lactic acidosis and renal failure. The absorption of organic acids of colonic bacterial origin can also contribute to this. Associated vomiting frequently exacerbates the acidosis by ECF contraction and lactic acidosis but can sometimes result in a primary metabolic alkalosis (Sect. 10.3), thus "normalizing" the pH.
Villous adenomas (usually of colon or rectum). They are potentially capable of malignant transformation.	May produce hypochloremic metabolic alkalosis (Sect. 10.9), but are equally capable (through uncertain mechanisms) of producing hyperchloremic acidosis. In the latter case,their secretions contain sodium and chloride of approximately the same concentration as in plasma. Severe fluid losses can sometimes ensue with circulatory shock and lactic acidosis.

9

Babior BM. Villous adenoma of the colon. Study of a patient with severe fluid and electrolyte disturbances. Am J Med. 1966;41:615–21.

Cieza J, Sovero L, Estremadoyro L. Electrolyte disturbances in elderly patients with severe diarrhea due to cholera. J Am Soc Nephrol. 1995;6:1463–7.

Gennari JF, Adrogue HJ, Galla JH, Madias NE. Acid base disorders and their treatment. Boca Raton: Taylor and Francis; 2005. p. 228–9.

Wang F, Butler T, Rabbani GH, Jones PK. The acidosis of cholera. Contributions of hyperproteinemia, lactic acidemia and hyperphosphatemia to an increased serum anion gap. N Engl J Med. 1986;315:1591–5.

9.35   Toxin Ingestion

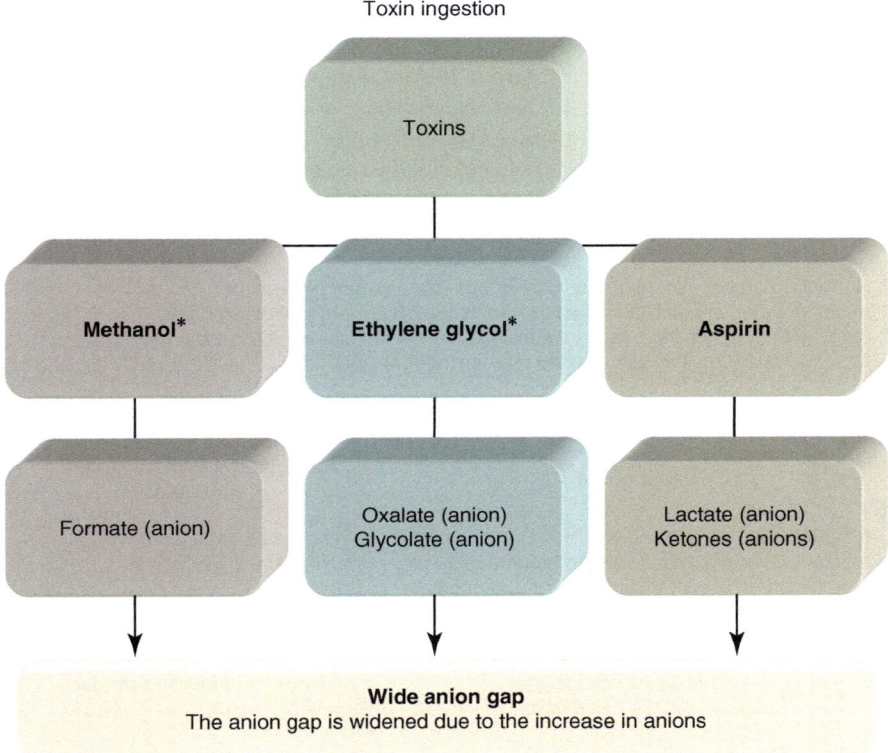

The first clue to the Methanol or Ethylene glycol poisoning is often the discovery of an osmolar gap (See Osmolar gap Sect. 9.41).

*The enzyme alcohol dehydrogenase helps in the catalysis of the reactions that lead to formation of the toxic metabolites. Co-ingested ethanol competes for the active sites on the enzyme alcohol dehydrogenase and so decreases the rate of formation of the methanol and ethylene glycol-induced toxic metabolites.

9

Post TW, Rose BD. Approach to the adult with metabolic acidosis. In: Basow DS, editor. UpToDate. Waltham: UpToDate; 2012. Last updated: 6 Oct 2010. Last accessed 13 May 2012.

9.36   Bicarbonate Gap (the Delta Ratio)

Syn: Delta gap, Delta-Delta gap, Deviation from the 1:1 correlation.

In wide anion gap metabolic acidosis, it is principally the decrease in the bicarbonate that accounts for the increase in the anion gap. If the decrease in the bicarbonate is disproportionate to the decrease in the anion gap, this implies the presence of an additional acid-base disorder. The difference between the increase in the anion gap (ΔAG) and the decrease in the bicarbonate (ΔHCO_3^-) is termed the bicarbonate gap.

Normally, *increase in anion gap = decrease in the serum bicarbonate* (Note that the venous CO_2 reflects serum bicarbonate levels). For example, if the anion gap has increased by 8 mEq/L, the serum bicarbonate is also expected to fall by 8 mEq/L. Two exceptions are possible:

The increase in the anion gap significantly exceeds decrease in the bicarbonate	The decrease in the bicarbonate significantly exceeds the increase in the anion gap
If the bicarbonate (which is an indicator of metabolic events), has not fallen proportionately, a process that is contributing to a *relative increase in the bicarbonate* in anticipated, i.e., *associated metabolic alkalosis is present.*	*An associated narrow anion gap metabolic acidosis is present*
Positive bicarbonate gap $\Delta AG - \Delta HCO_3^- > +6$ mEq/L	*Negative bicarbonate gap* $\Delta AG - \Delta HCO_3^- < -6$ mEq/L

9

In a pure wide anion gap metabolic acidosis, the fall in the bicarbonate need not always exactly parallel the rise in the AG: although the bicarbonate is the principal extracellular buffer, it is not the only buffer; there are other buffer systems that are also participating in the buffering process.

Martin L. All you really need to know to interpret arterial blood gases. Philadelphia: Lippincott Williams and Wilkins; 1999.

Wren K. The delta %) gap: an approach to mixed acid-base disorders. Ann Emerg Med. 1990;19:1310.

9.37   Urinary Anion Gap

A useful tool in narrowing down the cause of a hyperchloremic acidosis is the urinary anion gap.

Anions in the urine	Cations in the urine
• HCO_3^-	• Na^+
• Cl^-	• K^+
• PO_4^-	• Mg^{++}
• SO_4^-	• Ca^{++}
• Organic anions	• NH_4^{++}

Measured anions	Unmeasured anions	Measured cations	Unmeasured cations
Of these anions, only Cl^- is measured.	• HCO_3^- • PO_4^- • SO_4^-	Of the cations, only Na^+ and K^+ are measured.	• Mg^{++} • Ca^{++} • $NH4^{++}$

$$[Cl^-] + [UA]^* = [Na^+] + [K^+] + [UC]^{**}$$

i.e., the total no of anions equal the total no of cations, as per the law of electroneutrality.

Or,

$$UA - UC = [Na^+] + [K^+] - [Cl^-]$$

The urinary anion gap $= [Na^+] + [K^+] - [Cl^-]$

*Unmeasured Anions **Unmeasured Cations

9

The rationale for the use of UAG:

The concentration of *unmeasured anions* in the urine usually remains fairly *constant*. In some situations (e.g. the bowel-associated causes of NAGMA, Type 2 RTA), the output of $NH4^+$ *(the major unmeasured cation)* increases substantially.

$$UAG = UA - UC$$

The value of UAG therefore becomes negative. In effect, the UAG serves as a useful estimate of urine NH_4^+.

Battle DC, Hizon M, Cohen E, Gutterman C, Gupta R. The use of the urinary anion gap in the diagnosis of hyperchloremic metabolic acidosis. New Eng J Med. 1988;318:594–9.

9.38   Utility of the Urinary Anion Gap

The UAG helps distinguish between the principal causes of hyperchloremic acidosis. Most often the diagnosis is clinically apparent, and a calculation of the UAG is not generally necessary to make the distinction.

HCO₃⁻ loss from the bowel (as in diarrhea and Type 2 RTA)	HCO₃⁻ loss from the kidney (as in Types 1 and 4 RTA)
The renal response: excretion of H⁺. (Note that in Type 2 RTA the distal acidification of urine is normal).	The kidneys cannot increase H⁺ excretion
NH_4 concentration in the urine rises.	NH_4 concentration in the urine does not rises.
Negative UAG UAG = UA – UC Therefore, An increased UC will cause the value of UAG to be negative.	_No increase in UC: Positive UAG_ The value of UA – UC remains unchanged. UAG does not fall and retains its usual positive value. _(Abbreviation: UA = Urinary anions, UC = Urinary cations)._
A negative UAG in a hyperchloremic metabolic acidosis suggests bowel loss of bicarbonate (or Type 2 RTA).	A positive UAG in a hyperchloremic metabolic acidosis suggests renal loss of bicarbonate

The UAG may be misleading in neonates, as well as in the following:

Volume depletion as in diarrhea. (Ur Na⁺ < 25 mEq/L)	Compensatory increase in Cl⁻ reabsorption leads to decreased excretion of NH_4 (as NH_4Cl). This impairs distal acidification, simulating type 1 RTA.
Ketoacidosis (surplus unmeasured anions (ß-hydroxybutyrate and acetoacetate)	The excretion of the surplus unmeasured anions (ß-hydroxybutyrate and acetoacetate) requires co-excretion of Na⁺ and K⁺ to maintain electro-neutrality. Increased Ur Na⁺ and K⁺ can make the UAG positive _in spite of_ increased excretion of NH_4. $$UAG = Na^+ + K^+ - Cl^-$$

Battle DC, Hizon M, Cohen E, Gutterman C, Gupta R. The use of the urinary anion gap in the diagnosis of hyperchloremic metabolic acidosis. New Eng J Med. 1988;318:594–9.

9.39   Osmoles

> **Osmole:**
>
> The amount of substance that in an ideal solution, would yield the number of particles (Avogadro's number) that would depress the freezing point of solvent by 1.86K.

> **The usual circulating solutes in the body are:**
>
> Sodium (as chloride and bicarbonate salts)
> Glucose
> Urea

Under normal circumstances	**Under abnormal circumstances**
(when no circulating solutes other than sodium bicarbonate and urea are present):	*(in the presence of other measurable solutes in the circulation):*
Using a formula that takes into account the concentration of the above solutes, *the calculated value of these solutes will equal their measured value.*	*The measured value of the solutes will exceed the calculated value,* because the calculation does not take into account entities other than sodium, urea and glucose

9

9.40 Osmolarity and Osmolality

Osmolality

Osmolality is the number of osmoles of solute per **kilogram** of solvent. It is the osmotic activity in relation to the weight of the solvent.

- Osmolality is expressed in mOsm/kg of solute

- It is measured in the lab by osmometers.

Osmolarity

The number of osmoles of solute per litre of solvent. It is the osmotic activity in relation to the volume of the solvent.

- Omolarity is expressed in mOsm/L.

- It is a calculated value.

Several formulae for the calculation of plasma osmolarity are available
- $(2 \times Na) + glucose/18 + BUN/2.8$
- $(2 \times Na) + glucose/18 + BUN/2.8 + 9$
- $(2 \times Na) + glucose/18 + BUN/2.8 + Ethanol/4.6$

| The factor of 2 is on account of the chloride that accompanies the Na^+. | 2.8 is the conversion factor for glucose (for the conversion of mg/dL to mmol/L 0. | 18 is the conversion factor for blood urea nitrogen (for the conversion of mg/dL to mmol/L 0. |

9

Rose BD, Post TW. In: Clinical Physiology of Acid-Base and Electrolyte Disorders, 5th ed, McGraw-Hill, New York, 2001, p. 607–609.

Warhol RM, Eichenholz A, Mulhausen RO. Osmolality. Arch Intern Med. 1965;116:743.

9.41   Osmolar Gap

- The extent by which the measured value of solutes (osmolality) exceeds the calculated value of solutes (osmolarity) is termed the osmolar gap.
- *Synonyms: Osmolal gap, osmolarity gap, osmole gap*

- Osmolar gap = measured osmolality − calculated osmolarlity

- Since the values of osmolality (mOsm/L) and osmolarity (mOsm/L) are different (Sect. 9.40), they should ideally not be combined in the same equation.
- However, in clinical practice, this difference can usually be ignored, since in biological fluids the amount of solvent (water) is far in excess of the electrolyte particles.

9

Gennari FJ. Serum osmolality. Uses and limitations. N Engl J Med. 1984;301:102.

9.42   Abnormal Low Molecular Weight Circulating Solutes

With normal levels of solutes, e.g., Na + 140 mEq/L, Glucose 90 mg/dL and Blood urea nitrogen 14 mg/dL, the (calculated) plasma osmolality:

$$(2 \times 140) + 90 / 18 + 14 / 2.8 = 290 \text{ mOsm/L.}$$

Under normal circumstances, Na$^+$, glucose and urea are the only solutes present in any significant concentration. In the absence of additional solutes, the *measured* Osmolality will approximate the *calculated* Osmolarity, i.e., 290 mOsm/kg.

In the presence of abnormal low molecular weight circulating solutes such as methanol, ethylene glycol, ethanol and isopropyl alcohol which can be encountered as exogenous toxins:

Osmolality increases	**Osmolarity remains the same**
This is because osmolality is a measure of particles in addition to sodium glucose and urea.	This is because the calculation for osmolarity takes into account only glucose urea and sodium, all of which remain unchanged.

Osmolality will exceed osmolarity, since, as mentioned, the calculated value does not factor in solutes other than Na$^+$, glucose and urea.

Osmolar gap increases.

The principal diagnostic value of osmolar gap lies in raising the possibility of poisoning by the above substances as a cause of a wide-anion gap metabolic acidosis. It is important to remember that the osmolar gap is not infallible in its applications*.

9

---

*Sweeney TE, Beuchat CA. Limitations of methods of osmometry: measuring the osmolality of body fluids. Am J Physiol. 1993;264:R469.

Walker JA, Schwartzbard A, Krauss EA, et al. The missing gap: a pitfall in the diagnosis of alcohol intoxication by osmometry. Arch Intern Med. 1986;146:1843.

9.43   Conditions That Can Create an Osmolar Gap

Although several conditions can widen the osmolar gap, the mechanism by which they do so remains uncertain. The probable mechanisms are given below:

Diabetic Ketoacidosis	Lactic acidosis	Alcoholic Ketoacidosis	Methanol and ethylene glycol poisoning
Lipolysis	Glyogenolysis leads to small (non lactate) breakdown products.	Acetone and its metabolites	When DKA, lactic acidosis and alcoholic KA are ruled out, poisoning by methanol and ethylene glycol becomes a strong possibility.

> All the above conditions will result in a widened osmolar gap. Therefore a widened osmolar gap only becomes of diagnostic importance when these conditions are ruled out.

Other (uncommon) causes of a widened osmolar gap

- Mannitol
- Isopropyl alcohol
- IV immune globulin given in maltose (patients in renal failure cannot properly metabolize maltose).
- Hyperlipidemia (Pseudohyponatremia: the measured plasma sodium concentration is spuriously low leading to an *apparent* increase in osmolar gap).

9

Gabow PA. Ethylene glycol intoxication. Am J Kidney Dis. 1988;11:277.

Glasser L, Sternglanz PD, Combie J, Robinson A. Serum osmolality and its applicability to drug overdose. Am J Clin Pathol. 1973;60:695.

Robinson AG, Loeb JN. Ethanol ingestion: commonest cause of elevated plasma osmolality? N Engl J Med. 1971;284:1253.

Sklar AH, Linas SL. The osmolal gap in renal failure. Ann Intern Med. 1983;98:481.

Reference

Singer RB, Hastings AB: An improved clinical method for the estimation of disturbances of the acid-base balance of human blood. Medicine. 1948;27:223–242.

9

Chapter 10
Metabolic Alkalosis

Contents

10

A. Hasan, *Handbook of Blood Gas/Acid-Base Interpretation*,
DOI 10.1007/978-1-4471-4315-4_10, © Springer-Verlag London 2013

10.1   Etiology of Metabolic Alkalosis

Metabolic alkalosis is the most common acid-base disorder in hospitalized patients. Metabolic alkalosis involves a net gain of base, or a net loss of acid from the extracellular fluid. Its genesis needs the presence of *both* initiating and maintenance factors. Of itself, an initating factor cannot *sustain* a metabolic acidosis. Maintenance factors impede the excretion of the surplus bicarbonate and result in *perpetuation* of the alkalosis.

Increased extracellular bicarbonate	
Net gain of bicarbonate	Net gain of bicarbonate from an endogenous source
	• Metabolism of keto-anions
	Net gain of bicarbonate from an exogenous source
	• Sodium bicarbonate infusion
	• Ingestion of bicarbonate in renal failure
	• Metabolism by liver of organic anions to bicarbonate:
	o Citrate in massive blood transfusion
	o Lactate
	o Acetate
Fluid and ion shifts producing a *relative* increase in extracellular bicarbonate	Volume contraction in the presence of a relatively preserved extracellular bicarbonate content.

Decreased extracellular hydrogen ions	
Renal loss of hydrogen ions	Diuretic use
	• Post hypercapnic
	• Primary mineralocorticoid excess states
Gastrointestinal loss of hydrogen ions	Vomiting
	Continuous nasogastric tube aspiration

Galla, JH. Metabolic alkalosis. J Am Soc Nephrol 2000;11:369.

Garella, S, Chang, BS, Kahn, SI. Dilution acidosis and contraction alkalosis: review of a concept. Kidney Int 1975; 8:279.

Hodgkin JE, Soeprono EF, Chan DM. Incidence of metabolic alkalemia in hospitalized patients. Intensive Care Med.1980;8:725.

Palmer, BF, Alpern, RJ. Metabolic alkalosis. J Am Soc Nephrol 1997;8:1462.

Perez, GO, Oster, JR, Rogers, A. Acid-base disturbances in gastrointestinal disease. Dig Dis Sci 1987; 32:1033.

10

10.2 Pathways Leading to Metabolic Alkalosis

Chloride loss:	*GI tract:* Vomiting or nasogastric aspiration, villous adenoma, chloridorrhea, gastrocystoplasty. *Kidney:* Chloruretic diuretics, severe K^+ depletion, posthypercapnia. *Skin:* Cystic fibrosis.
Potassium loss:	*Gut:* laxative abuse. *Kidney:* hyperaldosteronism (primary and secondary), other hypokalemic hypertensive syndromes, Bartter and Gitelman syndromes.
Base loading in presence of low GFR	Milk-alkali syndrome. Base loading in ESRD. Co-administration of nonreabsorbable antacids and cation-exchange resin (Sect. 10.3).
Miscellaneous	Post-hypercapnic states. Multiple citrate blood transfusions. Widespread bony metastases. Recovery from starvation.

10

Garella, S, Chazan, JA, Cohen, JJ. Saline-resistant metabolic alkalosis or "chloride-wasting nephropathy". Ann Intern Med 1970; 73:31.

Seldin DW, Jacobson H. On the generation, maintenance and correction of metabolic alkalosis. Am J Physiol 1983;245:F425–F432.

10.3   Maintenance Factors for Metabolic Alkalosis

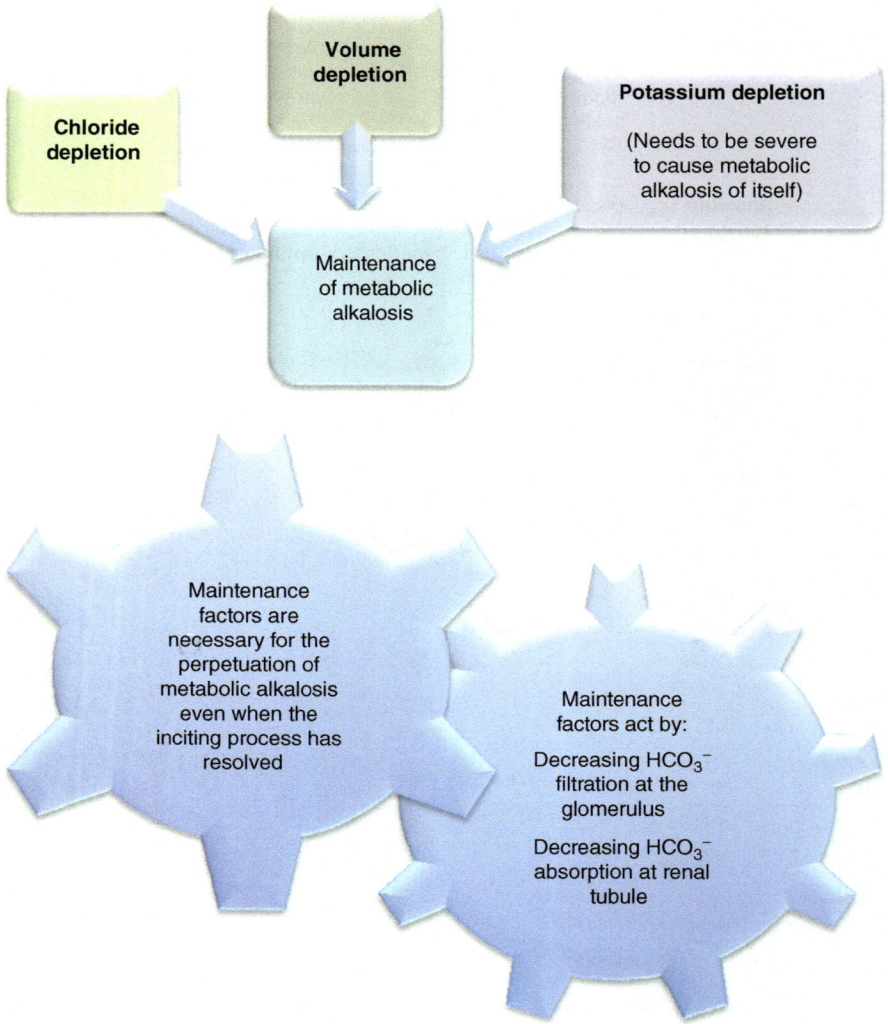

During the maintenance phase of chloride depletion metabolic alkalosis, urinary chloride levels are very low (or even absent) whereas in potassium depletion metabolic alkalosis urinary chloride levels are usually >20 mEq/L.

Berger BE, Cogan MG, Sebastian A. Reduced glomerular filtration rate and enhanced bicarbonate reabsorption maintain metabolic alkalosis in humans. Kidney Int. 1984;26:205.

Sabatini, S, Kurtzman, NA. The maintenance of metabolic alkalosis: Factors which decrease bicarbonate excretion. Kidney Int 1984; 25:357.

Seldin DW, Rector FC Jr. The generation and maintenance of metabolic alkalosis. Kidney Int 1972;1:306–321.

Luke RG, Wright FS, Fowler N, Kashgarian M, Giebisch G. Effects of potassium depletion on tubular chloride transport in the rat. Kidney Int 1978;14:414–427.

10.4   Maintenance Factors for Metabolic Alkalosis: Volume Contraction

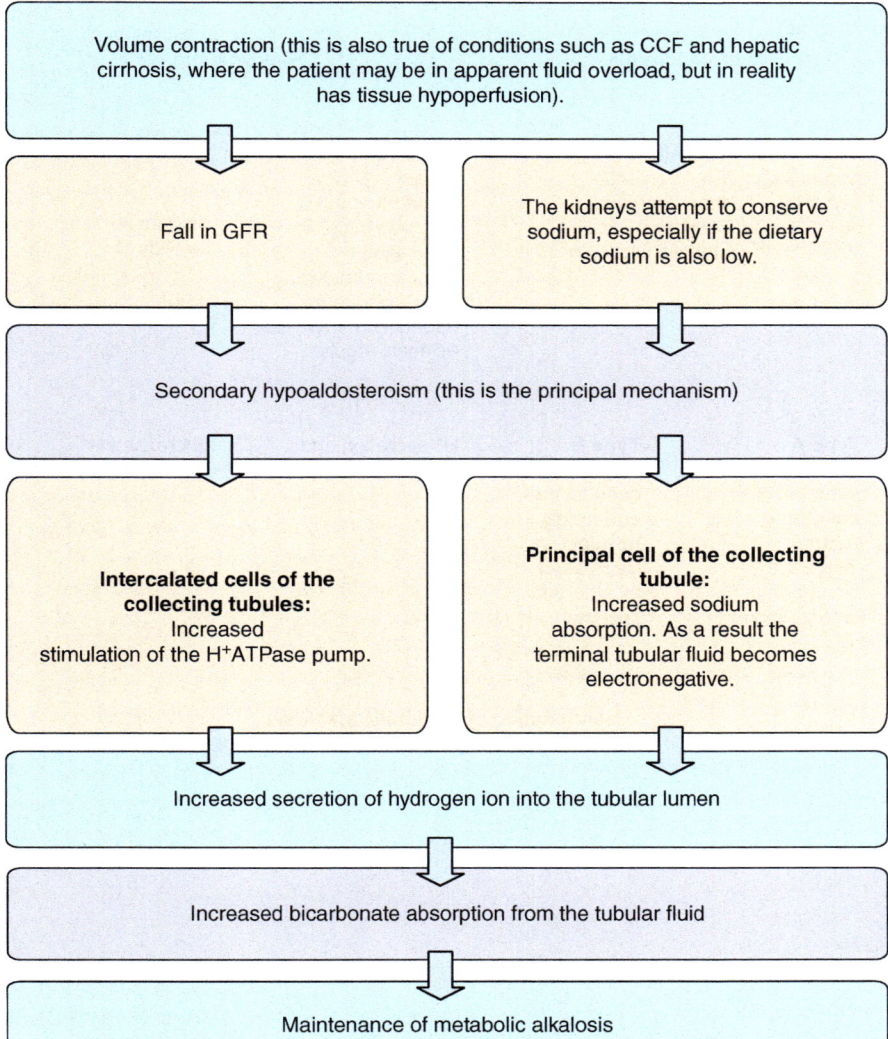

Berger BE, Cogan MG, Sebastian A. Reduced glomerular filtration rate and enhanced bicarbonate reabsorption maintain metabolic alkalosis in humans. Kidney Int. 1984;26:205.
Sabatini S, et al. 1984.

10.5   Maintenance Factors for Metabolic Alkalosis: Dyselectrolytemias

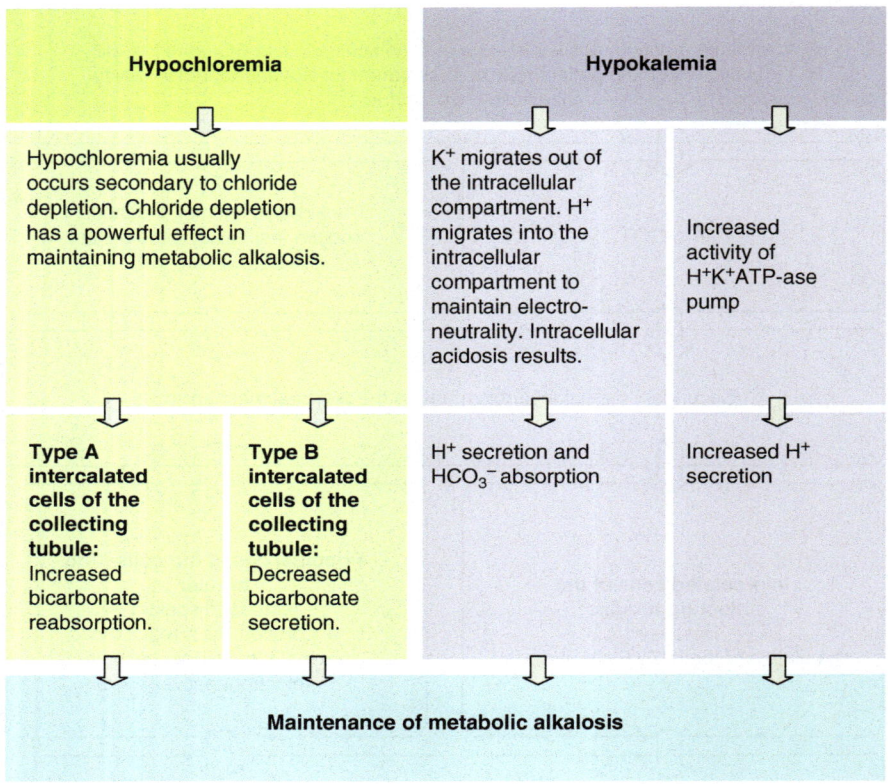

Galla, JH, Bonduris, DN, Luke, RG. Effects of chloride and extracellular fluid volume on bicarbonate reabsorption along the nephron in metabolic alkalosis in the rat. Reassessment of the classic hypothesis on the pathogenesis of metabolic alkalosis. J Clin Invest 1987;80:41.

Seldin DW, Jacobson H. On the generation, maintenance and correction of metabolic alkalosis. Am J Physiol 1983;245:F425–F432.

Wingo, CS, Smulka, AJ. Function and structure of H-K-ATPase in the kidney. Am J Physiol 1995;269:F1.

10.6   Compensation for Metabolic Alkalosis

Predicted PCO$_2$	ΔPCO$_2$
Predicted PCO$_2$ = (0.9 × HCO$_3^-$) + 9 ± 2. Alternatively, *Predicted PCO$_2$ = (0.7 × HCO$_3^-$) + 21* **Lower PCO$_2$** values than predicted indicate the presence of a coexisting respiratory alkalosis. **Higher CO$_2$** values than predicted indicate a coexisting respiratory acidosis.	The change in PCO$_2$ *(ΔPCO$_2$)* = (0.6–0.8) × ΔHCO$_3^-$

Of all the acid-base disorders, the confidence bands for the secondary respiratory response to metabolic alkalosis are the broadest (Sect. 10.9).

Limits of compensation for metabolic alkalosis

- The lungs are capable of hypoventilating such that the PCO$_2$ rises to a maximum of about 60 mmHg.

- PCO$_2$ levels in excess of this in primary respiratory acidosis may imply a coexistent primary metabolic alkalosis.

The "crossed anion" effect: Rarely (with excessive loss of Cl$^-$ as in prolonged vomiting or nasogastric aspiration), the plasma HCO$_3^-$ may exceed plasma Cl$^-$ levels, and the PaCO$_2$ may consequently increase beyond 60 mmHg. In such cases it is easy to misdiagnose and treat the metabolic acidosis as a respiratory acidosis.

10

Miller, PD, Berns, AS. Acute metabolic alkalosis perpetuating hypercapnia: A role for acetazolamide in chronic obstructive pulmonary disease. JAMA 1977; 238:2400.

Smith RM. In: Manual of clinical problems in pulmonary medicine. Ed: Bordow RA, Ries AL, Morris TA. Lippincott Williams and Wilkins. 6th ed 2005.

10.7   Urinary Sodium

Most of the time, the etiology of metabolic alkalosis is self-evident from the history. In more obscure cases, the analysis of urinary electrolytes may provide a clue.

Urinary sodium levels can differentiate hypovolemic from hypervolemic states

Urinary sodium <25 mEq/L	Urinary sodium >40 mEq/L
Implies sodium conservation i.e, hypovolemia	Implies absence of sodium conservation i.e., euvolemia

Urinary sodium may point to the broad etiology in unexplained metabolic alkalosis.

Hypovolemia (low urinary sodium)	Euvolemia or mild hyprvolemia (normal urinary sodium)
• Surreptitious vomiting as in bulimia • Surreptitious diuretic intake	• Mineralocorticoid excess states

Sometimes, for several reasons, urinary *sodium* may prove to be unreliable as an indicator of the subject's volume status, especially when there is significant bicarbonaturia (pH > 7.0). Urinary *chloride* estimation may more accurately reflect the patient's volume status (see next section).

10

Rose, BD. Clinical Physiology of Acid-Base and Electrolyte Disorders, 4th ed, McGraw-Hill, New York, 1994, pp. 522–530.

Sherman, RA, Eisinger, RP. The use (and misuse) of urinary sodium and chloride measurements. JAMA 1982; 247:3121.

10.8   Diagnostic Utility of Urinary Chloride (1)

Chloride-depletion alkalosis	Potassium-depletion alkalosis
Also called chloride-responsive alkalosis because it improves with Cl⁻ administration (as with NaCl infusion: *"saline responsive"*). It is the most common type of metabolic alkalosis.	Also known as chloride-resistant alkalosis: it is actually exacerbated when Cl⁻ is administered without K⁺ (e.g., NaCl infusion: *"saline unresponsive"*).
Hypokalemia and/or hypochloremia may be present.	Hypokalemia and/or hypochloremia may be present.
Urinary Cl⁻ <20 mEq/L (Often, urine Cl⁻ is<10 mEq/L).	**Urinary Cl⁻ >20 mEq/L.** A high urinary chloride suggests:

Chloride-depletion alkalosis

Also called chloride-responsive alkalosis because it improves with Cl^- administration (as with NaCl infusion: *"saline responsive"*). It is the most common type of metabolic alkalosis.

Hypokalemia and/or hypochloremia may be present.

Urinary Cl^- <20 mEq/L
(Often, urine Cl^- is<10 mEq/L).

Chloride depletion states:
GI tract: Vomiting or nasogastric aspiration, villous adenoma, chloridorrhea, gastrocystoplasty
Kidney: Chloruretic diuretics, severe K^+ depletion, posthypercapnia;
Skin: Cystic fibrosis.
However, urinary Cl^- is high when a chloriuretic diuretic is in use.
Post-hypercapnic states

Potassium-depletion alkalosis

Also known as chloride-resistant alkalosis: it is actually exacerbated when Cl^- is administered without K^+ (e.g., NaCl infusion: *"saline unresponsive"*).

Hypokalemia and/or hypochloremia may be present.

Urinary Cl^- >20 mEq/L.
A high urinary chloride suggests:

Ongoing diuretic therapy:
Decreased chloride absorption
Bartter's or Gitelman's syndrome
Severe hypokalemia (<2 mEq/L)
in potassium depletion states:
Gut: laxative abuse
Kidney: hyperaldosteronism, primary and secondary, other hypokalemic hypertensive syndrome, Bartter and Gitelman syndrome.

(Urine K^+ can be used to discriminate between these):

Urine K^+ <30 mEq/L reflects *severe* depletion of total body K^+ stores.	Urine K^+ >30 mEq/L reflects urinary K^+ wasting (mineralocorticoid excess or recent diuretic use).

10

Rose, BD. Clinical Physiology of Acid-Base and Electrolyte Disorders, 4th ed, McGraw-Hill, New York, 1994, pp. 522–530.

Sherman, RA, Eisinger, RP. The use (and misuse) of urinary sodium and chloride measurements. JAMA 1982; 247:3121.

10.9   The Diagnostic Utility of Urinary Chloride (2)

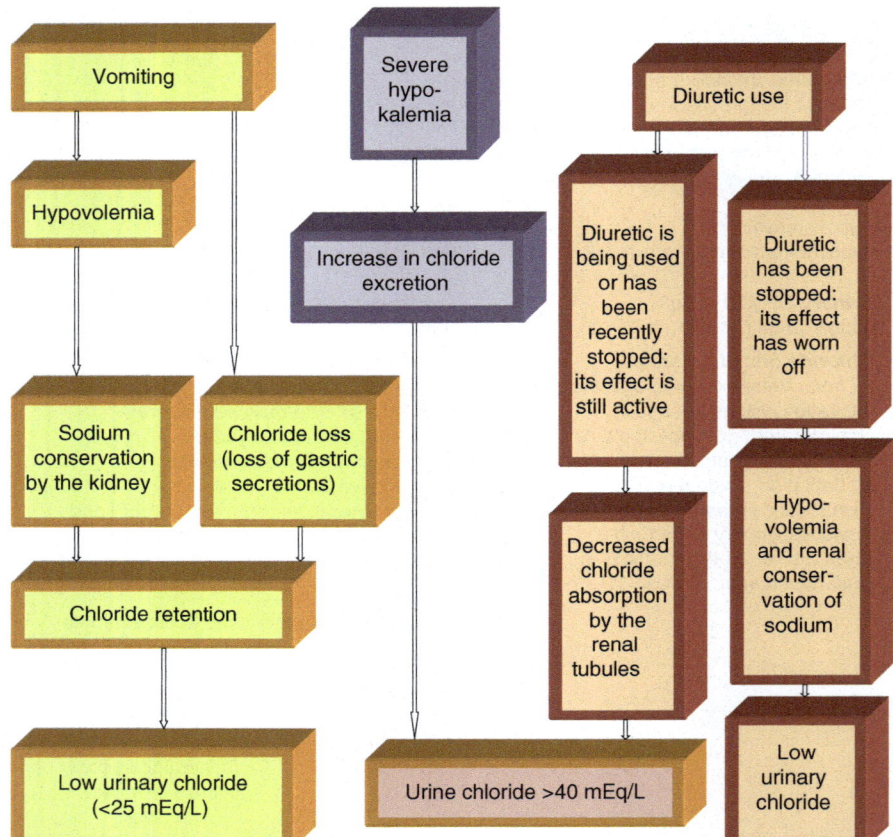

10.10   Diagnostic Utility of Urinary Chloride (3)

Volume contraction	Conservation of Na^+ and Cl^- by the kidney	Low urinary chloride
Vomiting	Loss of chloride-rich gastric secretions. Renal conservation of chloride	Hypochloremia Low urinary chloride
Prior diuretic therapy	There is an increase in the urinary chloride which is transient: urinary chloride levels gradually normalize when the diuretic is stopped.	Initially high followed by low urinary chloride
Cystic fibrosis	Loss of chloride in sweat Renal conservation of chloride	Hyperchloremia Low urinary chloride
Villous adenoma of the intestine	Diarrhea Loss of chloride into gut Renal conservation of chloride	Hyperchloremia Renal conservation of chloride Low urinary chloride
Post-hypercapnic metabolic alkalosis	Acute hypocapnia related chloride shifts	Low urinary chloride
Miscellaneous -Post-treatment for organic acidosis -Treatment with nonabsorbable anions (e.g., high doses of penicillin)		Low urinary chloride

A low urinary chloride indicates hypovolemia. In all the above cases, the chloride level is usually less than 25 mEq/L.

10

Garella, S, Chazan, JA, Cohen, JJ. Saline-resistant metabolic alkalosis or "chloride-wasting nephropathy". Ann Intern Med 1970;73:31.

Sherman, RA, Eisinger, RP. The use (and misuse) of urinary sodium and chloride measurements. JAMA 1982; 247:3121.

10.11   Some Special Causes of Metabolic Alkalosis

AGENT	MECHANISM
Vomiting	With frequent vomiting or continuous Ryle's tube drainage the acid-depleted gastric juice fails to evoke HCO_3^- excretion by the pancreas. The retained HCO_3^- leads to metabolic alkalosis.
Diarrhea	Loss of alkaline intestinal secretion from the body leads to the development of metabolic *acidosis*. Factitious diarrhea can cause metabolic *alkalosis* through unknown pathways.
Diuretics	Diuretics can produce metabolic alkalosis through multiple pathways: (1) *Volume depletion:* Secondary hyperaldosteronism and chloride depletion (2) *Potassium depletion* (3) *Chloride depletion:* Patients taking diuretics are also likely to be on a salt restricted (low chloride) diet; the kidney absorbs HCO_3^- to maintain electroneutrality. (4) *Loss of fixed acids* (anions). See also Sect. 10.5.
Alkali loading	Exogenous alkali intake (baking soda, citrate) or endogenous alkali generation (bone lysis) can result in metabolic alkalosis when the GFR is low (or if the intake is heavy, or if dietary salt intake [NaCl] is curtailed).
Penicillins (e.g. ampicillin)	"Non-reabsorbable" anionic antibiotics evoke K^+ and H^+ excretion through voltage effects in the collecting duct.
Hypo-albuminemia	The histidine groups of albumin contribute substantially to its buffering capacity. Hypoalbuminemia, consequently can produce a mild metabolic alkalosis
Hemodialysis	Citrate infusions are used in hemodialysis in lieu of heparin in those patients at risk of bleeding or those with heparin- induced thrombocytopenia. Since the calcium citrate cannot be excreted by the non-functioning kidneys, citrate-induced metabolic alkalosis can develop (it can be avoided by regulating the buffer content of the dialysate).
Cation exchange resins with antacids	Cations from antacids bind to the ingested cation-exchange resin. Bicarbonate, freed from the antacid is absorbed through the intestinal mucosa,but cannot be easily excreted in the setting of renal failure.

10

Brunner FP, Frick PG. Hypokalemia, metabolic alkalosis, and hypernatremia due to "massive" sodium penicillin therapy. Br Med J. 1968;4:550–2.

Cogan MG, Carneiro J, Tatsumo J. Normal diet NaCl variation can effect the renal set point for plasma pH- (HCO3) maintenance. J Am Soc Nephrol 1990;1:193–199.

Faber LM, de Vries PM, Oe PL, van der Meulen J, Donker AJ. Citrate haemodialysis. Neth J Med 1990;37:219–224.

10

Figge J, Rossing TH, Fencl V. The role of serum proteins in acid-base equilibria. J Lab Clin Med 1991;117:453–467.

Goidsenhoven GMT van, Gray OV, Price AV, Sanderson PH. The effect of prolonged administration of large doses of sodium bicarbonate in man. Clin Sci 1954;13:383–401.

Madias NE, Levey AS. Metabolic alkalosis due to absorption of "nonabsorbable" antacids. Am J Med 1983;74:155–158.

Marques MB, Huang ST. Patients with thrombotic thrombocytopenic purpura commonly develop metabolic alkalosis during therapeutic plasma exchange. J Clin Apheresis 2001;16:120–124.

Pinnick RV, Wiegmann TB, Diederich DA, Regional citrate anticoagulation for hemodialysis in the patient at high risk for bleeding . N Engl J Med 1983;308:258–261.

10.12   Metabolic Alkalosis Can Result in Hypoxemia

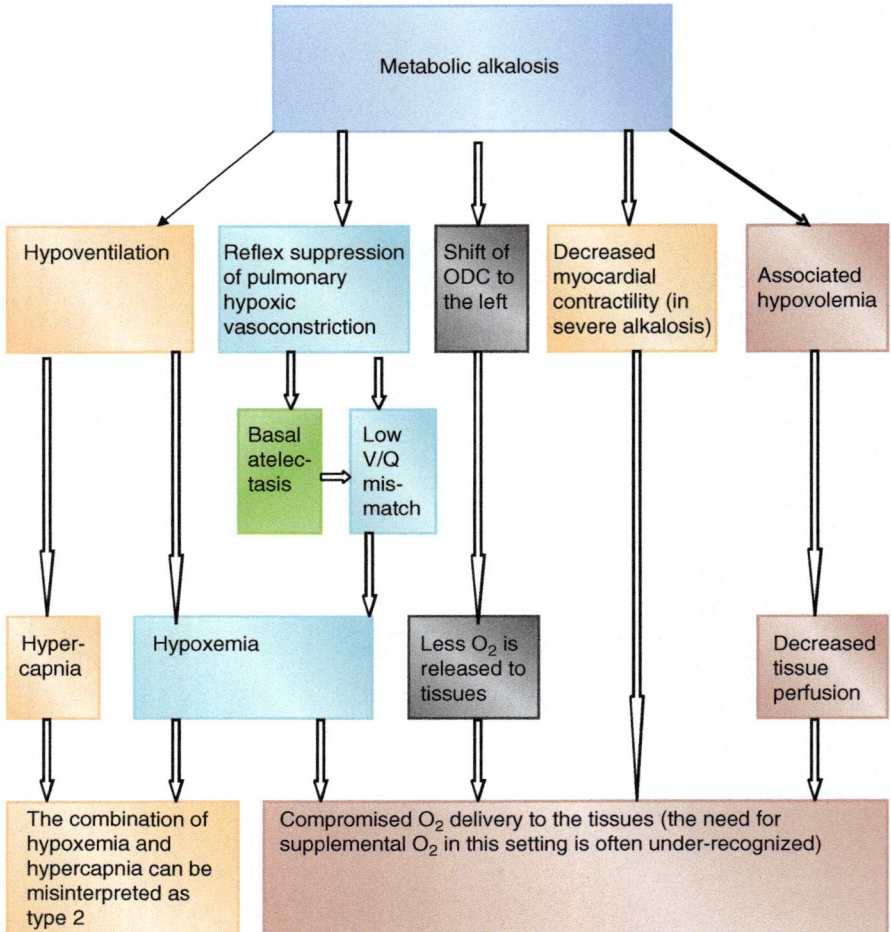

10.13   Metabolic Alkalosis and the Respiratory Drive

Metabolic alkalosis leads to compensatory hypoventilation

Hypoventilation results in hypoxemia

Became of the hypoxic stimulation of the respiratory drive, respiration cannot be depressed beyond a point. This limits the degree of compensation for the alkalosis.

When the PaO_2 falls to about 55 mmHg, the stimulus to breathe usually overcomes the respiratory depressant effect of the alkalosis.

Therefore the $PaCO_2$ cannot fall beyond a point.
When the $PaCO_2$ rises to above 60 mmHg, the following are possible:

Coexistent respiratory acidosis | Very severe metabolic alkalosis

See also "crossed anion" effect (Sect. 10.7).
Posthypercapnic metabolic alkalosis has been discussed under Sect. 7.8.

10

Bear R, Goldstein M, Phillipson E. Effect of metabolic alkalosis on respiratory function in patients with chronic obstructive lung disease. Can Med Assoc J. 1977;117:900–3.

Javaheri S. Compensatory hypoventilation in metabolic alkalosis. Chest 1982;81:296.

Javaheri S, Kazemi H. Metabolic alkalosis and hypoventilation in humans. Am Rev Respir Dis 1987;136:1101–1116.

Kilburn KH. Shock, Seizures, and Coma with Alkalosis During Mechanical Ventilation Ann Intern Med. 1 November 1966;65(5):977–984.

Pierce NF, Fedson DS, Brigham KL, et al. The ventilatory response to acute acid-base deficit in humans. Ann Intern Med 1970;72:633.

Chapter 11
The Analysis of Blood Gases

Contents

11

A. Hasan, *Handbook of Blood Gas/Acid-Base Interpretation*,
DOI 10.1007/978-1-4471-4315-4_11, © Springer-Verlag London 2013

11.1   Normal Values

	Arterial	Mixed Venous	Peripheral Venous
Partial Pressure of O_2	95–100 mmHg (PaO_2)	38–42 mmHg	40 mmHg
Saturation	>95 %	>70 %	65–75 %
Partial Pressure of CO_2	36–44 mmHg	44–46 mmHg	42–50 mmHg
Oxygen Content O_2/100 ml blood	~20 ml	~15 ml	~15 ml
pH	7.36–7.44	7.32–7.36	7.32–7.38
H^+	37–43 nEq/L		42–48 nEq/L
HCO_3^-	22–26 mEq/L	24–30 mEq/L	23–27 mEq/L

11.1.1   Venous Blood Gas (VBG) as a Surrogate for ABG Analysis

Under some circumstances, such as in ICUs or emergency rooms, it may be convenient to sample venous blood gases (VBGs). *Peripheral blood gases* can be sampled by standard venipuncture; *central venous blood gases* through central venous catheters; and *mixed venous blood gases* through the distal port of a pulmonary artery catheter (PAC). The latter are convenient to assess in a patient who has already had a PAC inserted. Central and mixed venous gases more closely reflect arterial gas measurements than do peripheral venous gases.

Venous pH, $PvCO_2$, and HCO_3^- are used to follow trends in the arterial pH, $PaCO_2$ and HCO_3^- respectively, provided there is no hemodynamic instability.

PvO_2 does not mirror PaO_2 in view of the fact that O_2 extraction by tissues occurs upstream to the venous sampling point.

11

Malatesha G, Singh NK, Bharija A, et al. Comparison of arterial and venous pH, bicarbonate, PCO_2 and PO_2 in initial emergency department assessment. Emerg Med J. 2007;24:569.

Malinoski DJ, Todd SR, Slone S, et al. Correlation of central venous and arterial blood gas measurements in mechanically ventilated trauma patients. Arch Surg. 2005;140:1122.

Middleton P, Kelly AM, Brown J, Robertson M. Agreement between arterial and central venous values for pH, bicarbonate, base excess, and lactate. Emerg Med J. 2006;23:622.

11.2   Step 1: Authentication of Data

Kassirer and Bleich's rule and the Henderson Hasselbach equation (see pH and H^+ equivalence) can be used to ascertain if the lab values obtained are reliable. A pH of 7.40 corresponds to a H^+ ion concentration of 40 nEq/L. Using Kassirer and Bleich's rule, a change in pH by 0.01 unit represents a change in H^+ ion concentration by 1 n Eq/L.

Is the following lab report authentic?
$$pH: 7.32, PCO_2: 32, HCO_3^-: 16.$$

The modified Henderson- Hasselbach equation:
$$H^+ = [24 \times CO_2]/HCO_3^-$$
Inserting the values of CO_2 and HCO_3^-,
$$H^+ = [24 \times 32]/16$$
$$H^+ = 48.$$

$H^+ = 48.$
This value represents an excess of 8 nEq/L over the normal (Normal H^+ level = 40 nEq/L).

Expected pH = $7.4 - [8 \times 0.01] = 7.32$
The data are authentic.

11

11.3   Step 2: Characterization of the Acid-Base Disturbance

Is the pH acidemic or is it alkalemic?	
Acidemia (pH < 7.36)	Alkalemia (pH > 7.44)

What is the source of the dominant acid-base disorder? *Is it Respiratory or is it Metabolic?*

Acidemia (pH < 7.36)	
Is a metabolic disturbance the cause for the acidemia (is the bicarbonate low?)	Is a respiratory disturbance the cause for the acidemia (is the $PaCO_2$ high?)
If yes, go to *METABOLIC TRACK.*	If yes, go to *REPIRATORY TRACK.*

Alkalemia (pH > 7.44)	
Is a metabolic disturbance the cause for the alkalemia (is the bicarbonate high?)	Is a respiratory disturbance the cause for the alkalemia (is the $PaCO_2$ low?)
If yes, go to *METABOLIC TRACK.*	If yes, go to *RESPIRATORY TRACK.*

11

11.4   Step 3: Calculation of the Expected Compensation

The compensation for respiratory disorders is by renal processes and vice versa. It is worth re-emphasising that interpretation of acid base disorders should always be made in the clinical context. If the compensation is less or more than expected, an *independent second disorder* exists.

Metabolic acidosis	*Compensation:* Expected $PaCO_2 = [1.5 \times HCO_3^-] + 8 \pm 4$ Alternatively, *change* in $PaCO_2 = 1.2 \times$ change in HCO_3^-
Metabolic alkalosis	*Compensation:* Predicted $PCO_2 = (0.7 \times HCO_3^-) + 21$ Alternatively, *change* in $PaCO_2 = 0.6^* \times$ change in HCO_3^-
Acute respiratory acidosis	Fall in pH = 0.008** $\times$ increase in $PaCO_2$. Alternatively, *Change* in $HCO_3^- = 0.1 \times$ change in CO_2
Chronic respiratory acidosis	Fall in pH = 0.003 $\times$ increase in $PaCO_2$. Alternatively, *Change* in $HCO_3^- = 0.4 \times$ change in CO_2
Acute respiratory alkalosis	Rise in pH = 0.01 $\times$ fall in $PaCO_2$*** Alternatively, *Change* in $HCO_3^- = 0.2 \times$ change in CO_2
Chronic respiratory alkalosis	Rise in pH = 0.003 $\times$ fall in $PaCO_2$ Alternatively, *Change* in $HCO_3^- = 0.5 \times$ change in CO_2

*0.6–0.8
**0.008 is virtually 0.01
***This relationship holds good for a $PaCO_2$ between 40 and 80 mmHg

To simplify this rather laborious method of acid-base analysis, I have integrated steps 2, 3 and 4 of this scheme into a single mnemonic-based method. I call it the Alpha-Numeric (a-1) approach (see Sect. 11.5)—AH

11

11.5   The Alpha-Numeric (a-1) Mnemonic

The alpha-numeric approach separates acid base disorders into one of two tracks depending on whether a metabolic or a respiratory process is responsible for the derangement. When an acid-base disorder is metabolic in origin the *METABOLIC TRACK* must be chosen. When an acid-base disorder is respiratory in origin, the *RESPIRATORY TRACK* must be chosen.

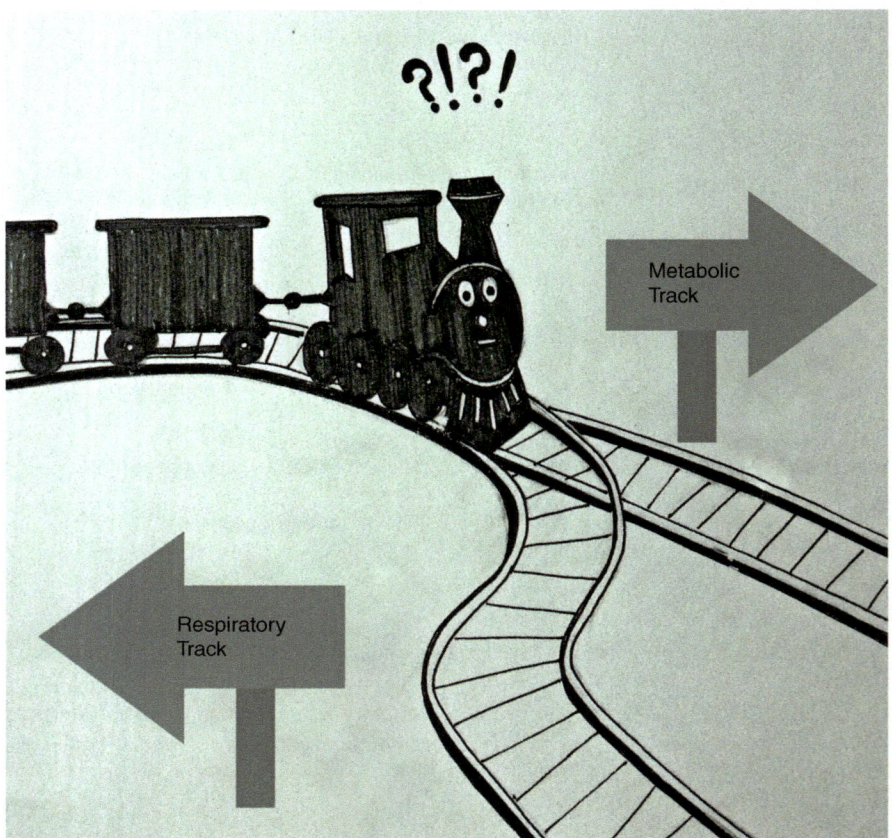

11

11.6   The Metabolic Track

If a metabolic process is the dominant cause of the acid-base derangement (i.e., if either metabolic acidosis or metabolic alkalosis is present), the metabolic approach must be chosen. Assessment of the A, B, and C components is relevant for metabolic acidosis, and assessment of D and E is relevant for metabolic alkalosis. In fact, assessment of the D component is relevant for *both* metabolic acidosis and metabolic alkalosis.

THE METABOLIC TRACK: A-B-C-D-E

A   *Anion gap*. Check the **Anion gap**. This helps narrow down the differential diagnosis.

B   *Bicarbonate gap:* ΔAG–ΔHCO_3
If > +6mEq/L, an associated metabolic alkalosis is present
If < +6mEq/L, an associated narrow-anion gap metabolic acidosis is present

C   *Colloid gap* (or, the Osmolar Gap):*
Measured osmolality minus calculated osmolarlity
Osmolarity: $(2 \times Na) + glucose/18 + BUN/2.8$
If the anion gap is wide (and DKA, lactic acidosis, uremia and salicylate poisoning have been ruled out), in the appropriate setting a *widened osmole gap provides a clue to toxin ingestion.*
For want of a better term I have called it a **Colloid gap (C--AH).*

D   *Disorder, associated primary respiratory:*

   (i)   If the primary condition is *Metabolic Acidosis* apply Winter's formula:

Predicted $PCO_2 = (1.5 \times HCO_3^-) + 8 \pm 2$

   (i)   If the primary condition is *Metabolic Alkalosis*:

Predicted $PCO_2 = (0.7 \times HCO_3^-) + 21 \pm 2$

E   *Electrolytes, urinary:*
Calculation of urinary anion gap (UAG) is relevant in hyperchloremic metabolic acidosis. *UAG = $[Na^+] + [K^+] - [Cl^-]$*
Negative UAG: bowel loss of bicarbonate
Positive UAG: renal loss of bicarbonate

11

11.7   The Respiratory Track

If a respiratory process is the dominant cause of the acid-base derangement (i.e., if either respiratory acidosis or respiratory alkalosis is present), the respiratory approach must be chosen. The box '**O**' pertains to oxygenation. *Only one* of the remaining four boxes should be chosen depending upon the clinical history (i.e., whether the presentation is *acute or chronic*) in the particular circumstance (respiratory *acidosis* or respiratory *alkalosis*). 0.**1**, 0.**2**, 0.**4** or 0.**5** are mnemonics for the relevant equations (see below).

THE RESPIRATORY TRACK: 0-1-2-3-4-5

O	*Oxygenation, assessment of:* PaO_2/FIO_2 ratio $(A-a)DO2$
0.1	*Acute respiratory acidosis:* The HCO_3^- increases by *0.1* mEq/l for every 1 mmHg rise in CO_2 $\Delta HCO_3^- = \Delta CO_2 \times 0.1$ Expected $HCO_3^- = 24 + \Delta HCO_3^-$
0.2	*Acute respiratory alkalosis:* The HCO_3^- decreases by *0.2* mEq/l for every 1 mmHg fall in CO_2 $\Delta HCO_3^- = \Delta CO_2 \times 0.2$ Expected $HCO_3^- = 24 - \Delta HCO_3^-$
0.4	*Chronic respiratory acidosis:* The HCO_3^- increases by *0.4* mEq/l for every 1 mmHg rise in CO_2 $\Delta HCO_3^- = \Delta CO_2 \times 0.4$ Expected $HCO_3^- = 24 + \Delta HCO_3^-$
0.5	*Chronic respiratory alkalosis:* The HCO_3^- falls by *0.5* mEq/l for every 1 mmHg fall in CO_2 $\Delta HCO_3^- = \Delta CO_2 \times 0.5$ Expected $HCO_3^- = 24 - \Delta HCO_3^-$

Δ = change in

*For me, the "0.3" in the mnemonic has no role in the mnemonic—yet (until you can think one up for it!)—AH

11.8   Step 4: The 'Bottom Line': Clinical Correlation

Lastly, it is imperative to correlate the results of the ABG analysis with the clinical condition of the patient. As in all other aspects of clinical medicine, the importance of the history and physical examination cannot be overemphasized: any interpretation of blood gases must be made in the appropriate clinical context. However for the purpose of brevity, clinical information has been truncated in the case histories to follow; an attempt at clinical correlation has been made at the end of each worked example.

When there is lack of correlation between the clinical picture and the ABG values, the blood gas report must be reviewed for possible ambiguities (see Sects. 13.1, 13.2, 13.3, 13.4, 13.5, 13.6 and 13.7).

11

11.8.1   Clinical Conditions Associated with Simple Acid-Base Disorders

CONDITION	ACID-BASE DISORDER
Vomiting	Metabolic alkalosis
Diarrhea	Metabolic alkalosis or Metabolic acidosis in severe secretory diarrhea (NAGMA)
Diuretic therapy	Metabolic alkalosis
Diabetic ketoacidosis	Metabolic acidosis (wide anion gap) at presentation. A normal anion gap metabolic acidosis often develops during therapy
Renal failure	Metabolic acidosis
Seizures	Metabolic acidosis (lactic) acidosis
Cyanide, CO poisoning	Metabolic (lactic) acidosis acidosis due to histotoxic hypoxia
Renal tubular acidosis	Metabolic acidosis (normal anion gap)
Hypotension, low cardiac output states, severe anemia.	Metabolic (lactic) acidosis
Biguanide, INH therapy	Metabolic acidosis (lactic) acidosis
Antibiotic therapy	Metabolic acidosis (D-lactic acidosis)
Cirrhosis	Respiratory alkalosis
Pregnancy	Respiratory alkalosis
Hypoxemia	Respiratory alkalosis or acidosis depending on whether there is type 1 or type 2 respiratory failure respectively. Metabolic (lactic) acidosis if hypoxemia severe.
Pneumonia (reflex hyperventilation)	Respiratory alkalosis
ALI/ARDS (reflex hyperventilation)	Respiratory alkalosis
Asthma exacerbation	Respiratory alkalosis (respiratory acidosis when respiratory muscle fatigue occurs)
Pulmonary thromboembolism	Respiratory alkalosis
Severe COPD; see also conditions listed under 'causes of hypoventilation' (Sect.1.35)	Respiratory acidosis

11

11.8.2   Mixed Disorders

Mixed disorders can be *additive* (two disorders, either both producing alkalemia, or both producing acidemia); alternatively, mixed disorders can be *counterbalancing* (with two disorders, one producing alkalemia and the other producing acidemia), for example:

CONDITION	ACID-BASE DISORDER
Cardiopulmonary arrest	Metabolic acidosis (lactic acidosis due to circulatory failure) + respiratory acidosis (respiratory arrest).
Cardiogenic shock with pulmonary edema	Metabolic acidosis (lactic acidosis due to circulatory failure and hypoxemia) + respiratory acidosis (hypoventilation due to pulmonary edema).
Chronic renal failure with superimposed respiratory failure	Metabolic acidosis (WAGMA of renal failure) + respiratory acidosis (superadded respiratory acidosis of any etiology—see Sects. 7.2 and 9.28).
Renal tubular acidosis with muscle weakness	Metabolic acidosis (NAGMA due to RTA) + respiratory acidosis (respiratory muscle fatigue due to hypokalemia)
Dyselectrolytemia with diarrhea	Metabolic acidosis (secretory diarrhea, which is the proximal cause of the hypokalemia) + respiratory acidosis (hypokalemia related respiratory muscle weakness).
Diabetic ketoacidosis with hypophosphatemia	Metabolic acidosis (WAGMA due to diabetic ketoacidosis) + respiratory acidosis (respiratory muscle fatigue due to hypophosphatemia + Kussmaul's breathing).
Severe vomiting in pregnancy	Metabolic alkalosis (hypochloremic alkalosis due to vomiting) + respiratory alkalosis (physiological hyperventilation of pregnancy).
Hepatic cirrhosis with vomiting	Metabolic acidosis (hypochloremic alkalosis due to vomiting) + respiratory alkalosis (chronic liver disease).
Hepatic cirrhosis with diuretic use	Metabolic alkalosis (diuretic) + respiratory alkalosis (chronic liver disease)
Ryle's tube drainage and sepsis	Metabolic alkalosis (hypochloremic metabolic alkalosis due to Ryle's tube drainage) + respiratory alkalosis (reflex tachypnea due to sepsis)

11

Septic shock	Metabolic acidosis (lactic acidosis) + respiratory alkalosis (reflex tachypnea).
Diabetic ketoacidosis and sepsis (eg, pneumonia)	Metabolic acidosis (diabetic ketoacidosis) + respiratory alkalosis (sepsis/pneumonia- related tachypnea).
Renal failure and pneumonia	Metabolic acidosis (WAGMA due to renal failure) + respiratory alkalosis (pneumonia - related reflex tachypnea).
Salicylate toxicity	Metabolic acidosis (possibly due to organic acids, but likely multifactorial; lactic acidosis accounts for the late component of salicylate- induced metabolic acidosis) + respiratory alkalosis (direct stimulation of respiratory centre by salicylate, uncoupling of oxidative phosphorylation in chemoreceptor cells).
Hepatorenal syndrome	Metabolic acidosis (of both renal and hepatic origin) + respiratory alkalosis (of hepatic origin).
Cor pulmonale treated with diuretics	Metabolic alkalosis (diuretic) + respiratory acidosis (chronic respiratory failure).
Chronic respiratory failure with vomiting	Metabolic alkalosis (hypochloremic alkalosis) + respiratory acidosis (pre-existing chronic respiratory disease)

11

Morganroth ML. An analytic approach to diagnosing acid-base disorders. J Crit Illn. 1990; 5(2):138–50.
Narins RG. Simple and mixed acid-base disorders: a practical approach. Medicine. 1980; 59:161–87.

11.9   Acid-Base Maps

Acid-base maps offer an alternative (and quick!) way of interpreting compensatory responses to simple acid-base disorders. They are also useful in confirming that the "compensatory" changes are physiologically possible. It is not possible to diagnose "triple disorders" (two metabolic disturbances with one of the respiratory disorders) by acid base mapping.

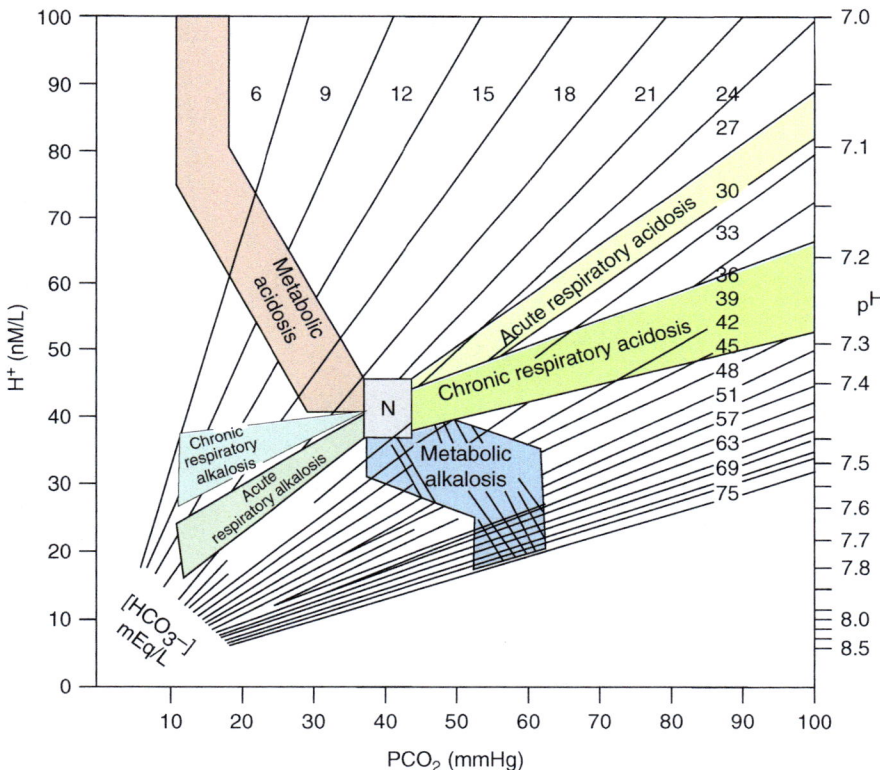

On the ordinate, the blood H± concentration (in nanomoles/L) is given on the left; the pH is given on the right. On the abscissa is represented the PCO_2 (in millimetres of mercury). The diagonal lines running across the map are the isopleths for blood HCO_3 concentration (in mEq/L). Within the box in the centre of the map falls the range of normal values. Six bands diverge from this box, each representing the 95 % confidence limits for a simple acid-base disorder.

When a given patient's values fall upon any such band, a simple acid-base disorder corresponding to that band may be presumed: it is however not mandatory that a simple acid base disorder exists in such a patient. When the values fall outside any of the bands a mixed acid-base disturbance is very likely.

11

Goldberg M, Green SB, Moss ML, et al. Computer-based instruction and diagnosis of acid-base disorders: a systematic approach. JAMA. 1973;223:269–75.

Chapter 12
Factors Modifying the Accuracy of ABG Results

Contents

12

A. Hasan, *Handbook of Blood Gas/Acid-Base Interpretation*,   267
DOI 10.1007/978-1-4471-4315-4_12, © Springer-Verlag London 2013

12.1   Electrodes

Arterial blood gases (ABGs) are necessary for the investigation, monitoring and clarification of mechanisms of gas exchange, and of acid–base disorders. The design of the electrodes in the blood gas analyser is based on the model of the electro-chemical cell. Two half-cells are immersed in an electrolyte solution. An external connection which includes an ammeter, completes the circuit. Chemical reactions that consume electrons occur at each half-cell in solution. The half-cell at which the stronger of the two reactions occurs, becomes the cathode; the other half cell (which is therefore negative relative to the first half-cell) becomes the anode.

The temperature of the chamber is held constant: usually at 37 °C. The chemical reactions produce a measurable flow of electrons through the external circuit.

The blood is analysed by three separate electrodes (see opposite page). Most blood gas machines *measure* pH and PCO_2 but rather *calculate* HCO_3^- from the Henderson-Hasselbach equation using pH and PCO_2. This of course means that examination of the pH and PCO_2 alone conveys the greatest part of the information contained within the ABG printout.

O_2 electrode (The Clark electrode)	The working of the O_2 electrode is based on the principle of polarography. The electrode includes a silver anode and a platinum cathode immersed in potassium chloride solution. A semi-permeable membrane separates this solution from the blood sample. O_2 molecules diffuse into the cell and react with the cathode. The number of electrons produced by this reaction is proportional to the pO_2 of the blood sample.
pH electrode (The Sanz electrode)	Compared to the Clark electrode, the Sanz electrode is complex. The essence of this electrode is a special hygroscopic glass membrane. The glass membrane separates the blood sample from an electrolyte solution. The membrane is kept completely hydrated. On contact with the blood sample, hydrogen ions dissociate from the membrane and produce a measurable flow of electrons. A current is generated within the electrode depending upon this difference in the electrical charges on either side.
CO_2 electrode (The Severinghaus electrode)	The CO_2 electrode is a glass electrode immersed in a bicarbonate buffer solution. The latter is contained in a nymlon spacer and separated by a membrane from the blood sample. CO_2 diffuses out of the blood sample, through the silicone membrane and into the bicarbonate buffer solution, altering the pH of the latter. The H^+ are measured by a modified pH cell. The difference in the electrical potential creates a current. The number of hydrogen ions generated within the bicarbonate solution is proportional to the PCO_2.

12

Hansen JE. Arterial blood gases. In: Mahler DA, editor. Pulmonary function testing. Clin Chest Med. 1989;5:227–37.

Madama, VC. In: Pulmonary Function Testing and Cardiopulmonary Stress Testing, 2nd ed., Delmar, 1998.

12.2   Accuracy of Blood Gas Values

With improvements in technology, the confidence limits for all values are very narrow.

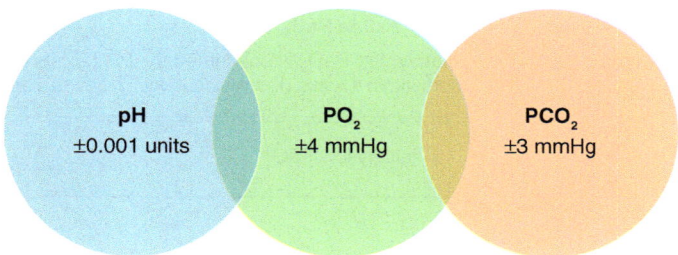

12

Glauser FL, Morris JF. Accuracy of routine arterial puncture for the determination of oxygen and carbon dioxide tensions. Am Rev Respir Dis. 1972;106:776.

12.3   The Effects of Metabolizing Blood Cells

Metabolizing cells in the blood contained within the syringe consume O_2

Fall in PaO_2
If the syringe is not iced immediately, the PaO_2 is consumed by the blood cells in the sample (if a sample can be analysed within 15 min of drawing it, icing may not be required*)

falsely low PaO_2

*Hansen JE. Arterial blood gases. In: Mahler DA, editor. Pulmonary function testing. Clin Chest Med. 1989;5:227–37.

12.4 Leucocyte Larceny

> Abnormally high number of leukocytes or thrombocytes (e.g., leukemia or thrombocytosis) can consume a large amount of O_2 in spite of icing the sample.

> Falsely low PaO_2 ("pseudohypoxemia")

Because the pseudohypoxemia often persists despite prompt icing and analysis of the sample, another mechanism may be operative.

> The leucocytes and thrombocytes may coat the surface of the electrode.

> This possibly physically impedes the O_2 from gaining access to the electrode.

> Promptly centrifugation of the blood upon drawing the sample and analysis of the supernatant plasma prevents this problem.

Charan NB, Marks M, Carvalho P. Use of plasma for arterial blood gas analysis in leukemia. Chest. 1994;105:954–5.

Hess CE, Nichols AS, Hunt WB, et al. Pseudohypoxemia secondary to leukemia and thrombocytosis. N Engl J Med. 1979;301:361–3.

12

12.5   The Effect of an Air Bubble in the Syringe

The effect of an air bubble on the arterial blood in a syringe can have a variable effect on the PaO_2, and a predictable effect on the pH and the $PaCO_2$. The gases in the blood sample and in the trapped air bubble will, by the process of diffusion, tend to equilibrate with each other over time.

PaO_2	The PaO_2 of ambient air at sea level is approximately 160 mmHg, so this is the PaO_2 of an air bubble trapped within a syringe.	If the PaO_2 of the arterial blood is <160 mmHg, the measured PaO_2 will rise.
		If the PaO_2 of the arterial blood is >160 mmHg, the measured PaO_2 will fall.
$PaCO_2$	CO_2 is present in miniscule levels in ambient air. In other words the $PaCO_2$ in a trapped air bubble is virtually zero.	The $PaCO_2$ of the arterial blood will trend towards zero, no matter what its initial value.
pH	The effect of the trapped air bubble on the pH is related to its effect on the $PaCO_2$.	As the $PaCO_2$ of the blood falls due to the effect of the air bubble, pH will rise, i.e, the blood will become more alkalemic

12

Mueller RG, Lang GE, Beam JM. Bubbles in samples for blood gas determinations: a potential source of error. Am J Clin Pathol. 1976;65:242.

12.6   Effect of Over-Heparization of the Syringe

Heparin is a sulfated mucopolysaccharide with acidic properties. An excess of heparin in the ABG syringe can have the following effects:

Effect on pH	Dilutional effect

If the pH is *normal or alkaline* to begin with:	If the pH is *very acidic* to begin with:	
		The PaO$_2$ and PaCO$_2$ can also be spuriously lowered by dilution.
Acidemia increases	**Acidemia decreases**	
pH will fall on contact with the acidic heparin.	pH will rise as the mildly acidic heparin reduces the greater acidity of the blood.	

12

12.7   The Effect of Temperature on the Inhaled Gas Mixture

Due to the humidifying effect of the upper airways, inhaled gas is completely saturated with water vapour: the partial pressure of water vapour in the inhaled air is 47 mmHg.

Pyrexia	Hypothermia
The partial pressure of water vapor rises to slightly above 47 mmHg	The partial pressure of water vapor falls to slightly below 47 mmHg
As a result, the partial pressure of the remaining gases, cumulatively, falls to slightly below 713 mmHg (760 minus [>47] mmHg)	As a result, the partial pressure of the remaining gases, cumulatively, rises to slightly above 713 mmHg (760 minus [<47] mmHg)

However, the actual change in the above figures is too small to make a clinical difference.

12

Bacher A. Effects of body temperature on blood gases. Intensive Care Med. 2005;31:24.
Shapiro BA. Temperature correction of blood gas values. Respir Care Clin N Am. 1995;1:69.

12.8   Effect of Pyrexia (Hyperthermia) on Blood Gases

In clinical practice, the contribution of temperature to the measurement of blood gases is not considered important*. There is usually little change in the SpO_2 and CaO_2 with a change in temperature***

Pyrexia (>39 °C)	O_2 in a febrile patient (esp >39 °C):	Decreased solubility of O_2 in the blood with a rise in temperature.	Over-estimation of hypoxemia	For every degree C over 37° rise in the patient's temperature, the PO_2 should be increased by 7.2 % (PaO_2 will be shown about 5 mmHg lower than it actually is).
	CO_2 in a febrile patient (esp >39 °C):	Decreased solubility of CO_2 in the blood with a rise in temperature.	Under-estimation of acidosis.	For every degree C over 37° rise in the patient's temperature, the PCO_2 should be decreased by 4.4 % ($PaCO_2$ will be shown about 2 mmHg lower than it actually is).
	pH in a febrile patient	As the temperature of the body rises, the pH falls.	Over-estimation of pH.	For every degree C over 37° rise in the patient's temperature, the pH should be decreased by 0.015 units.

Curley FJ, Irwin RS. Disorders of temperature control: part I. Hyperthermia. J Int Care Med. 1986;1:5.

*Hansen JE, Sue DY. Should blood gas measurements be corrected for the patient's temperature? N Engl J Med. 1980;303:341.

***Severinghaus JW. Oxyhemoglobin dissociation curve correction for temperature and pH variation in human blood. J Appl Physiol. 1958;12:485–6.

12

12.9   Effect of Hypothermia on Blood Gases

Hypo-thermia	O_2 in a hypo-thermic patient:	Increased solubility of O_2 in the blood with a fall in temperature.	Under-estimation of hypoxemia.	For every degree C below 37° fall in the patient's temperature, the PO_2 should be decreased by 7.2 % (PaO_2 will be shown about 5 mmHg higher than it actually is).
	CO_2 in a hypo-thermic patient:	Increased solubility of CO_2 in the blood with a fall in temperature.	Over-estimation of acidosis.	In vitro changes in acid-base status parallel those in vivo: correction of PCO_2 is not required.
	pH in a hypo-thermic patient:	As the temp-erature of the body falls, the pH rises.	Under-estimation of pH.	In vitro changes in acid-base status parallel those in vivo: correction of pH is not required.

Bacher A. Effects of body temperature on blood gases. Intensive Care Med. 2005;31:24.

Curley FJ, Irwin RS. Disorders of temperature control: part I. Hyperthermia. J Int Care Med. 1986;1:5.

Rahn H, Reeves RB, Howell BJ. Hydrogen ion regulation, temperature, and evolution. Am Rev Respir Dis. 1975;112:165–72.

Shapiro BA. Temperature correction of blood gas values. Respir Care Clin N Am. 1995;1:69.

12.10   **Plastic and Glass Syringes**

Plastic syringes	Glass syringes
• O_2 can diffuse out of plastic syringes, especially at high PaO_2's (e.g., >221 mmHg). This can spuriuosly lower the measured PaO_2. • Also, excessive suction force is often required with plastic syringes, especially if the patient's blood pressure is low (<70 mmHg). This can pull gas out of solution, lowering the PaO_2 by as much as 12 mmHg.	• Glass syringes are less pervious to O_2. • PaO_2 will be more or less unaltered for up to 3 h* in an iced sample of blood contained within a glass syringe.

Ansel GM, Douce FH. Effect of needle syringe material and needle size on the minimum plunger-displacement pressure of arterial blood gas syringes. Respir Care. 1982;27:127.

*Canham EM. Interpretation of arterial blood gases. In: Parsons PE, Weiner-Kronish JP, editors. Critical care secrets. 3rd ed. Philadelphia: Hanley and Belfus, Inc.; 2003. p. 21.

Winkler JB, Huntington CG, Wells DE, Befeler B. Influence of syringe material on arterial blood gas determinations. Chest. 1974;66:518.

12

Chapter 13
Case Examples

Contents

A. Hasan, *Handbook of Blood Gas/Acid-Base Interpretation*,
DOI 10.1007/978-1-4471-4315-4_13, © Springer-Verlag London 2013

13

The First Critical Step

The first critical step in the evaluation of a blood gas sample is the bringing forth of a detailed history. The importance of a reliable history cannot be overemphasized. From the history, a shortlist of the differential diagnoses is constructed, and the ABG sample is interpreted against this background.

However, in the examples to follow, the history has been deliberately abbreviated, and a clinical correlation has been attempted at the end of the analysis. In these examples, the algorithmic approach presented throughout this volume has been adhered to. Acid base maps (see Sect. 11.9) are presented on the facing page to enable familiarity with both methods.

13

13.1   Patient A: A 34 year-old man with Metabolic Encephalopathy

A 34 year old man presents to ER and is worked up for a possible metabolic encephalopathy. His blood gases are as follows:

pH 7.31, $PaCO_2$ 26 mmHg, PaO_2 94 mmHg, Na^+: 138 mEq/L, K^+: 4.0 mEq/L, Cl^-: 103 mEq/L, HCO_3^-: 18 mEq/L

The object of this example is the importance of verification of data. Regardless of the history, the ABG sample must be analyzed for internal consistency; if there is lack of internal consistency, the authenticity of the reported values becomes questionable.

We knnow that:

$$[H^+] = 24 \times PaCO_2/HCO_3^-$$

The equivalent values for $[H^+]$ and pH are as follows (Sect. 3.10):

pH	$[H^+]$
7.6	25
7.5	32
7.4	40
7.3	50
7.2	63
7.1	79
7.0	100

$$[H^+] = 24 \times 26/18$$

$$[H^+] = 34.7$$

However the pH is about 7.3, aand for that pH the H^+ should be 50. The data are inconsistent.

13

13.2   Patient B: A 40 year-old man with Breathlessness

A 40 year old breathless man is found to have a PaO_2 of 65 mmHg on room air. Supplemental oxygen is administered by nasal prongs, and a blood gas sample half an hour later reveals a PaO_2 of 100 mmHg. How much increase in the oxygen content of the blood has been produced by increasing the FIO_2?

Answer: virtually none. At a PaO_2 of 65 mmHg, the SpO_2 By increasing the FIO_2, the hemoglobin, fully saturated as it is, is not capable of being saturated any further. The CaO_2 therefore remains unaltered on this account. The increase in FIO_2 does result in a small increment in *dissolved* O_2, but since the amount of dissolved O_2 is relatively the tiny, the enhancement in the CaO_2 is negligible.

13

13.3   Patient C: A 50 year-old woman with Hypoxemia

A 50 year old woman is found to have a PaO_2 of 50 mmHg on room air. Supplemental oxygen is administered, and her PaO_2 rises to 100 mmHg. What is the change in the oxygen content of the blood given that his hemoglobin is 15 gm/dL?

Assuming no shift in the position of the oxy-hemoglobin dissociation curve, a PaO_2 of 50 mmHg corresponds approximately to a SpO_2 of 85 %, and a PaO_2 of 100 mmHg to 98 %.

$CaO_2 = 1.34 \times SpO_2 \times Hb$ (see Sect. 1.23)

CaO_2 on room air

$CaO_2 = 1.34 \times 0.85 \times 15$

$CaO_2 = 17$ mL O_2/dL.

CaO_2 on supplemental oxygen

$CaO_2 = 1.34 \times 0.98 \times 15$

$CaO_2 = 19.7$ mL O_2/dL.

The CaO_2 has increased by about 14 %.

The effect that a fall in Hb has on the CaO_2 can be profound. Looking at the equation:

$$CaO_2 = 1.34 \times SpO_2 \times Hb$$

It can be appreciated that a fall in the Hb produces a fall in CaO_2 of the same order of magnitude. For example if the Hb were to drop to half of its original value (to 7.5 g/dL from 15 g/dL), the drop in CaO_2 would also be by 50 % (see also 'Patient P' later).

13

13.4   Patient D: A 20 year-old woman with Breathlessness

A 20 year old woman with no previous medical problems was brought to the hospital complaining of breathlessness. She had a PaO_2 of 118 mmHg and a $PaCO_2$ of 20 mmHg on room air.

A rule of the thumb is that on room air, the sum of the PaO_2 and the $PaCO_2$ should add up to about 140, which it does in this case ($118 + 20 = 138$).
This makes an underlying mechanism of hypoxemia unlikely.

A more sensitive test for a defect in oxygenation is the $A\text{-}aDO_2$, which is of course the partial pressure of O_2 in the alveolus (PAO_2) minus the partial pressure of oxygen in the arterial blood (PaO_2).

$$A\text{-}aDO_2 = PAO_2 - PaO_2.$$
$$PAO_2 = FIO_2\,(Pb - Pw) - PaCO_2/R$$

Assuming a barometric pressure of 760 mmHg (sea level),
and a respiratory quotient of 0.8:

$$PAO_2 = [0.21\,(760 - 47)] - (20/0.8)$$

$PAO_2 = 149 - 25$

$PAO_2 = 124$

$A\text{-}aDO_2 = PAO_2 - PaO_2 = 124 - 118$

$A\text{-}aDO_2 = 6$ (Normal $A\text{-}aDO_2$ is <14 on room air)
The $A\text{-}aDO_2$ is normal.

The patient gave a history of emotional turmoil. Subsequent evaluation did not turn up pulmonary thromboembolism or any other problem.

13

13.5   Patient E: A 35 year-old man with Non-resolving Pneumonia

Diagnostic bronchoscopy for a non-resolving pneumonia has just been completed in a 35 year old non-smoker, when his SpO_2 is seen to fall to 88 % in spite of administration of 2L of oxygen per minute by nasal prongs. The patient had tolerated the bronchoscopy with a satisfactory SpO_2 on the same liter-flow of O_2 a few minutes ago. An ABG reveals a PaO_2 of 110 mmHg.

The PaO_2 seems slightly low for the FIO_2 being given. 2 litres per minute on nasal prongs are the equivalent of an FIO_2 of about 0.28. This would result in a PaO_2 of about 140 mmHg in a normal individual (28 × 5). In the clinical context, a mild V/Q mismatch post-bronchoscopy, and possibly the pneumonia itself, could account for a PaO_2 which is slightly lower than expected from the calculation.

A PaO_2 of 110 mmHg, however, certainly does not agree with a SpO_2 of 88 %.

The clinical setting is compatible with local-anaesthetic induced methemoglobinemia, and co-oximetry should be used to confirm the diagnosis.

13

13.6   Patient F: A 60 year-old man with Cardiogenic Pulmonary Edema

The SpO_2 of a 60 year old man recovering in the ICU from an acute coronary syndrome, has fallen to 86 % on supplemental oxygen. The chest X-ray shows possible mild interstitial pulmonary edema.

pH 7.43 HCO_3: 24 mEq/L, $PaCO_2$: 37 mmHg, PaO_2 126 mmHg on 35 % oxygen by ventimask.

The PaO_2 seems slightly low for the FIO_2 being given, but can be accounted for by the recumbency and possible mild cardiogenic pulmonary edema. What is interesting is the disparity between the PaO_2 and SpO_2. The ABG shows no obvious acid-base disorder.

The clinical setting is that of an acute coronary artery syndrome, and it is safe to assume that the patient is on nitrates; the latter are commonly implicated in the genesis of methemoglobinemia.

Methemoglobinemia was later confirmed on co-oximetry.

13.7 Patient G: A 72 year-old Drowsy COPD Patient

A 72 year old COPD patient was brought to the EMD. During transport, Mr. G had been given oxygen supplementation by a partial rebreathing mask at 12 l/min. At reception, Mr. G was drowsy and was breathing at only 5–6 breaths/min. An ABG performed on arrival showed pH 7.19, PaO_2 66 mmHg, $PaCO_2$ 92 mmHg.

Treatment options would include:

(a) Administering FIO_2 at 0.28 by ventimask
(b) Making the patient breathe room air to augment the his hypoxic ventilatory drive
(c) Increasing FIO_2 by administering O_2 through a non-rebreathing mask

The correct answer is (a). It is conceivable that the high flow oxygen administered to the patient during transport has suppressed his respiratory drive, compounding the hypercapnic respiratory failure. Reducing the FIO_2 to an acceptable level is logical, in that the patient would still be getting enough FIO_2 to maintain a reasonable O_2 saturation and the reduction in FIO_2 would also enhance the patient's hypoxic respiratory drive, thereby increasing his minute ventilation.

Many physicians may feel that it would be premature to intubate and ventilate the patient in a situation such as this, and would rather give the patient a chance to recover with a trial of initial conservative therapy. Noninvasive positive pressure ventilation in this setting is important despite the potential risk of aspiration in a drowsy patient: it may help avert invasive mechanical ventilation. Bronchodilators, corticosteroids, antibiotics and respiratory stimulants may be used as the situation demands, with recourse to mechanical ventilation being taken if the PaO_2 is not sustainable at >60 mmHg with conservative therapy, or if there is a progressive rise in $PaCO_2$ with acidosis in spite of optimal treatment.

Completely stopping supplemental oxygen is *not* an option. The PAO_2 (the partial pressure of oxygen in the alveolus) is determined by the following equation:

$$PAO_2 = \left[(P_{atm} - P_w) \times FIO_2 \right] - \left[(PaCO_2/RQ) \right]$$

Where,
PAO_2 = Partial pressure of oxygen in the alveolus
P_{atm} = Atmospheric pressure (760 mmHg at sea level)
P_w = Partial pressure of water vapour (47 mmHg)
FIO_2 = Fractional concentration of O_2 (delivered oxygen)
$PaCO_2$ = Partial pressure of carbon dioxide
RQ = Respiratory Quotient (taken as 0.8 in this example)

Thus, at sea level, assuming that 12 (LPM) by partial rebreathing mask corresponds to an FIO_2 of approximately 0.6,

$$PAO_2 = \left[(760 - 47) \times 0.6 \right] - \left[(92/0.8) \right] = 312.8 \text{ mmHg}$$

13

If the supplemental O_2 were to be suddenly stopped, the patient would be breathing room air only ($FIO_2 = 0.21$) and with a PCO_2 of 92 mmHg,

$$\mathbf{PAO_2} = \left[(760 - 47) \times 0.21 \right] - \left[(92/0.8) \right] = 34 \text{ mmHg}$$

A low partial pressure of oxygen in the alveolus would mean that the arterial PaO_2 would be lower yet, and this could result in cerebral hypoxia.

Supplemental oxygen should therefore never be completely stopped.

Adapted from: Hasan A. Understanding Mechanical Ventilation: A Practical Handbook. London: Springer; 2010. Case 11. p. 522–3.

13

13.8   Patient H: A 30 year-old man with Epileptic Seizures

History:

A 30 year old man is brought to the ER with a recent epileptic seizure.
pH: 7.19 HCO$_3^-$: 18 mEq/L, PCO$_2$: 48 mmHg

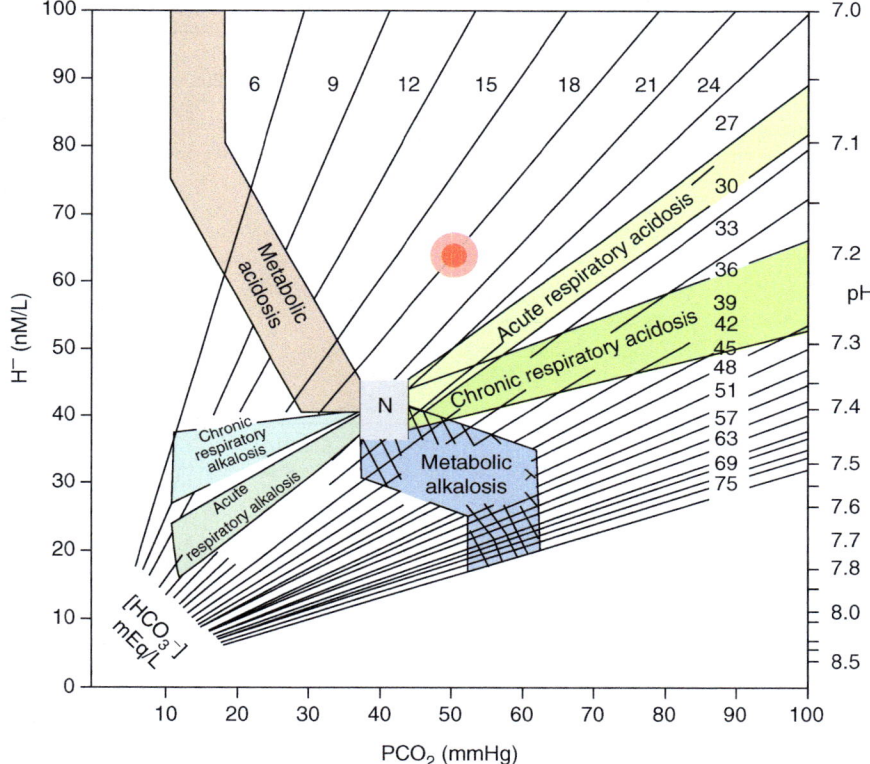

Patient H

This patients values fall on a point midway between the "95 % confidence bands"
of acute respiratory acidosis and metabolic acidosis. Both acute respiratory acidosis
and metabolic acidosis are likely to be present.

13

pH: Acidemic	
Is metabolic acidosis the cause of the acidemia (is the bicarbonate low?)	Is respiratory acidosis the cause of the acidemia (is the $PaCO_2$ high?)
Yes	Yes

It is evident that there is a mixed acidosis: both metabolic and respiratory acidoses coexist, and it is unnecessary to look for 'associated' primary acid-base disorders.

THE METABOLIC TRACK: A-B-C-D-E	
A	*Anion gap*: In most cases of metabolic acidosis, it is relevant to know the status of the anion gap. In this example, though, the data necessary for the calculation of the anion gap have not been furnished.
B	*Bicarbonate gap: $\Delta AG - \Delta HCO_3^-$* *If > +6 mEq/L, an associated metabolic alkalosis is present* *If < +6 mEq/L, an associated narrow-anion gap metabolic acidosis is present*
C	*Colloid gap: Measured osmolality minus calculated osmolarlity* Osmolarlity: $(2 \times Na^+)$ + glucose/18 + BUN/2.8 If the anion gap is wide (and DKA, lactic acidosis, uremia and salicylate poisoning have been ruled out), in the appropriate setting a *widened osmole gap provides a clue to toxin ingestion.*
D	*Disorder, associated primary respiratory:* (i) If the primary condition is *Metabolic Acidosis* apply Winter's formula: Predicted $PCO_2 = (1.5 \times HCO_3^-) + 8 \pm 2$ (i) If the primary condition is *Metabolic Alkalosis*: Predicted $PCO_2 = (0.7 \times HCO_3^-) + 21 \pm 2$
E	*Electrolytes, urinary:* Calculation of urinary anion gap (UAG) is relevant in hyperchloremic metabolic acidosis. *UAG = $[Na^+] + [K^+] - [Cl^-]$* *Negative UAG: bowel loss of bicarbonate* *Positive UAG: renal loss of bicarbonate*

Clinical Correlation:
The hypoventilation (respiratory acidosis) is consistent with a recent seizure. So is the metabolic acidosis, presumably due to hyperlactatemia, which can be expected to be a wide-anion gap one.

13

13.9   Patient I: An Elderly Male with Opiate Induced Respiratory Depression

An elderly male presents to the ER with opiate induced respiratory depression. pH 7.19, HCO_3^-: 20 mEq/L, PCO_2: 56, PaO_2: 115 on supplementary O_2.

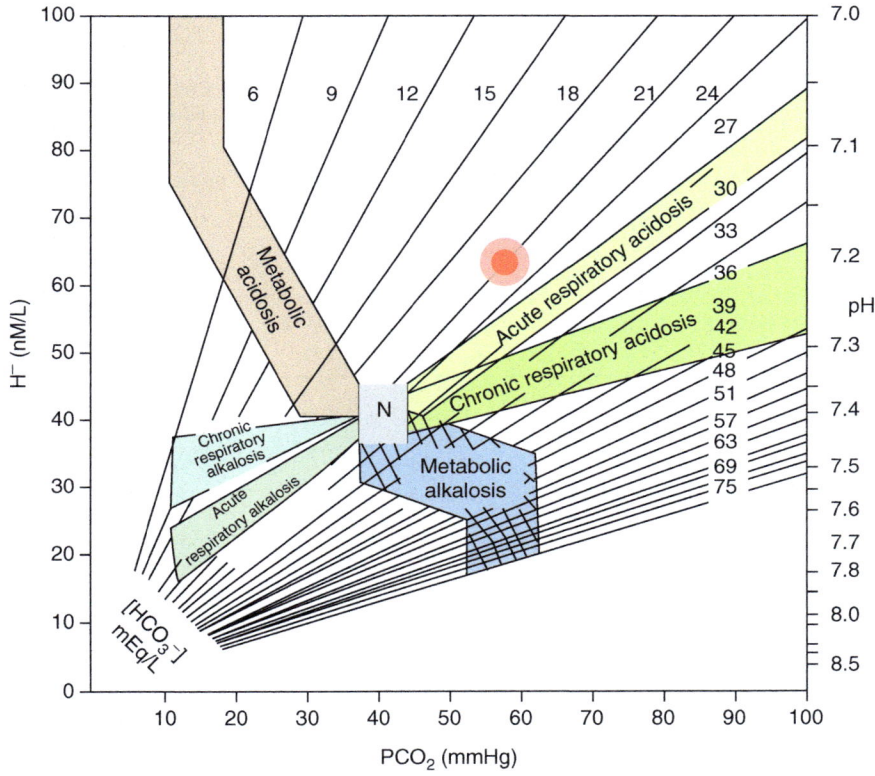

Patient I

As in the previous example, the patient's values fall on a point midway between the bands of acute respiratory acidosis and metabolic acidosis. Both acute respiratory acidosis and metabolic acidosis are therefore likely to be present.

13

pH 7.19: Acidemia	
Is metabolic acidosis present (is the bicarbonate low?)	Is respiratory acidosis present (is the $PaCO_2$ high?)
Yes. Apply the METABOLIC A-B-C-D-E TRACK	Yes.

It is evident that there is a mixed acidosis: both metabolic and respiratory acidoses coexist, and it is unnecessary to look for 'associated' primary acid-base disorders.

THE METABOLIC TRACK: A-B-C-D-E	
A	*Anion gap*: In this example data to calculate the anion gap has not been provided, but the anion gap needs to be calculated to further characterize the metabolic acidosis.
B	*Bicarbonate gap:* The bicarbonate gap (delta ratio) also needs to be calculated to further characterize the metabolic acidosis (as will be shown in examples further on).
C	*Colloid gap: Measured osmolality minus calculated osmolarlity* Osmolarlity: $(2 \times Na)$ + glucose/18 + BUN/2.8 If the anion gap is wide (and DKA, lactic acidosis, uremia and salicylate poisoning have been ruled out), in the appropriate setting a *widened osmole gap provides a clue to toxin ingestion.*

D	*Disorder, associated primary respiratory:*
	    (i) If the primary condition is *Metabolic Acidosis* apply Winter's formula:
	Predicted $PCO_2 = (1.5 \times HCO_3^-) + 8 \pm 2$
	
	    (i) If the primary condition is *Metabolic Alkalosis*:
	Predicted $PCO_2 = (0.7 \times HCO_3^-) + 21 \pm 2$

E	*Electrolytes, urinary:* Calculation of urinary anion gap (UAG) is relevant in hyperchloremic metabolic acidosis. *$UAG = [Na^+] + [K^+] - [Cl^-]$* *Negative UAG: bowel loss of bicarbonate* *Positive UAG: renal loss of bicarbonate*

The Clinical correlation
The respiratory acidosis is clearly due to respiratory depression by the sedative. A cause for the metabolic acidosis needs to be sought.

13

13.10 Patient J: A 73 year-old man with Congestive Cardiac Failure

A 73 year old man on diuretic therapy presented to the ER in congestive cardiac failure.

pH 7.62 PCO_2 35 mmHg, PO_2 70 mmHg, HCO_3^- 32 mEq/L, K^+ 2.3 mEq/L, Normal anion gap, Urinary spot chloride 72 mEq/L.

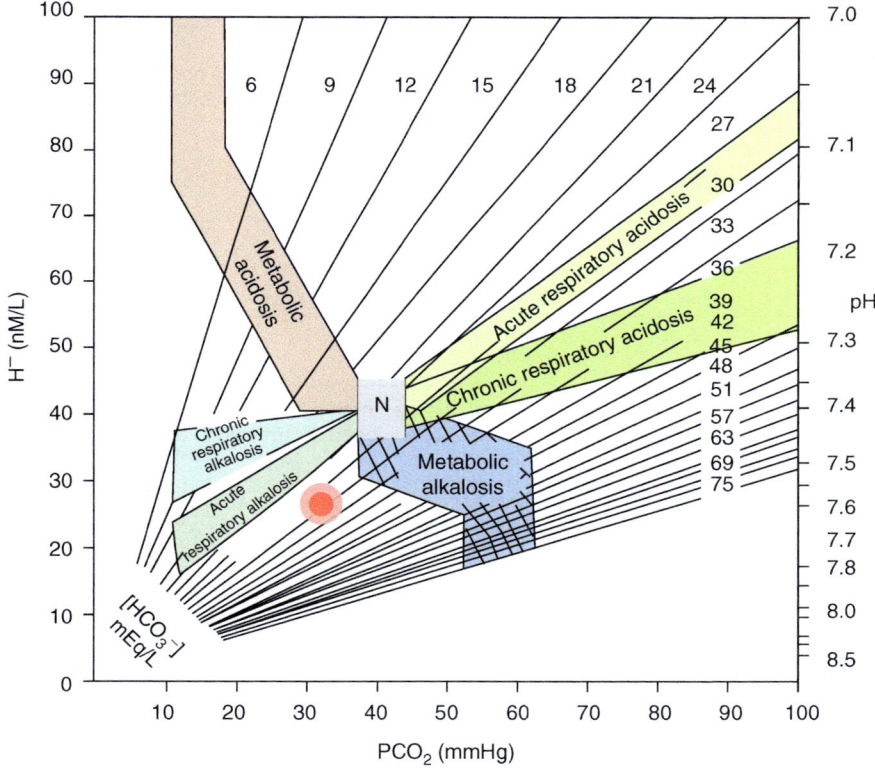

Patient J

This patients values fall on a point between the bands of acute respiratory alkalosis and metabolic alkalosis. Acute respiratory alkalosis and metabolic alkalosis are both likely to be present.

13

pH 7.64: Alkalemia	
Is metabolic alkalosis the cause of the alkalemia (is the bicarbonate high?)	Is respiratory alkalosis the cause of the acidemia (is the $PaCO_2$ low?)
Yes. Apply the METABOLIC A-B-C-D-E TRACK	Yes. The CO_2 as noted, is low when it should be high, so a primary respiratory alkalosis is also present**

It is evident that there is a mixed alkalosis: both metabolic and respiratory alkaloses coexist, and it is unnecessary to look for 'associated' primary acid-base disorders.

THE METABOLIC TRACK: A-B-C-D-E	
A	*Anion gap (AG):* Since the primary disorder is metabolic alkalosis, the anion gap is not of direct relevance. However an unexpectedly wide anion gap is sometimes the only clue to a coexistent metabolic acidosis. $AG = Na^+ - (Cl^- - HCO_3^-)$ That the anion gap is normal, and there is no metabolic acidosis*** has already been mentioned.
B	*Bicarbonate gap: $\Delta AG - \Delta HCO_3$* *If > + 6 mEq/L, an associated metabolic alkalosis is present* *If < + 6 mEq/L, an associated narrow-anion gap metabolic acidosis is present*
C	*Colloid gap: Measured osmolality minus calculated osmolarlity* Osmolarlity: (2x Na) + glucose/18 + BUN/2.8
D	*Disorders (respiratory) associated with the metabolic alkalosis:* An associated respiratory alkalosis has already been determined to be present based on (discussions) above
E	*Electrolytes (urine):*The urinary spot sodium (72) is elevated, which is consistent with a chloride-resistant metabolic alkalosis*

Clinical correlation:
*The patient has been using diuretics which are a common cause of chloride-resistant metabolic alkalosis
**The respiratory alkalosis is due to the hyperventilation due to the CCF
**Hypoxemia and a reduced organ perfusion due to CCF could produce a lactic acidosis which is a HAGMA. However, in this case, there is no metabolic acidosis

13

13.11   Patient K: A 20 year-old woman with a Normal X-ray

A 20 year old woman is under evaluation in the ER for acute shortness of breath. Her chest X-ray is interpreted as normal:

pH: 7.55, HCO_3^-: 22 mEq/L, PCO_2: 27 mmHg, PO_2: 93 mmHg on room air. The anion gap is normal.

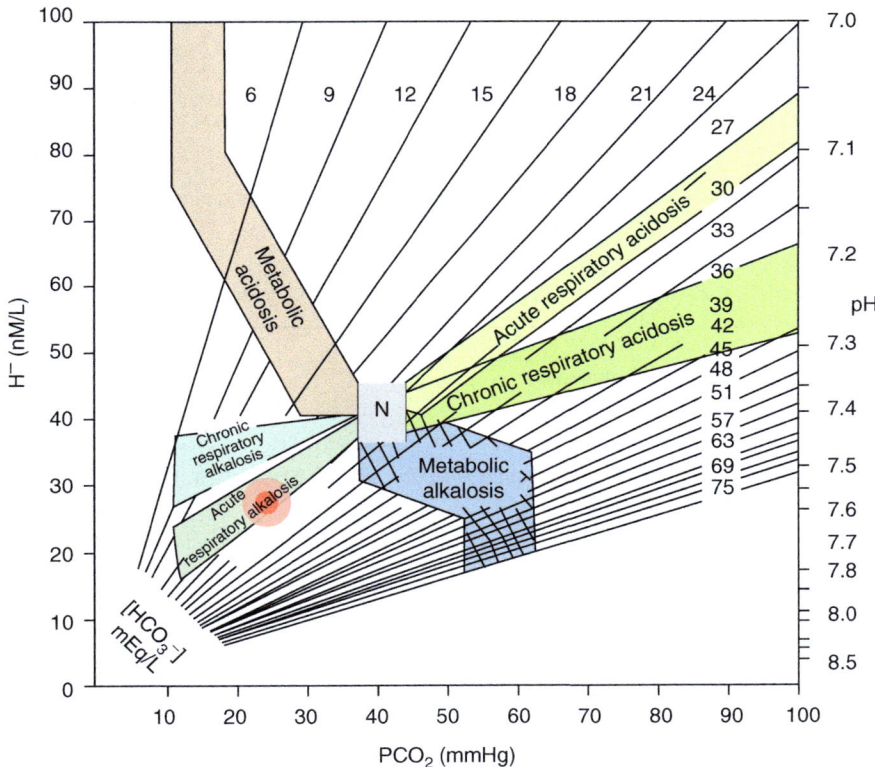

Patient K

The patient's values fall on the band of acute respiratory alkalosis. As mentioned in Sect. 11.9, when a patient's values fall on any of the "95 % confidence bands", a simple acid-base disorder is likely to be present (in this case, acute respiratory alkalosis).

13

pH 7.55: Alkalemia	
Is metabolic alkalosis present (is the bicarbonate high?)	Is respiratory alkalosis present (is the $PaCO_2$ low?)
No.	Yes.
(Also, the anion gap: given as normal. No associated metabolic acidosis is present).	**Is an associated metabolic disorder present?** Apply the formula for acute Respiratory alkalosis

	THE RESPIRATORY TRACK: 0-1-2-(3)-4-5 (Block 2 is relevant here)
O	**Oxygenation:** The PaO_2 is 93 mmHg on an FIO_2 of 0.21 (should be: $0.21 \times 5 = 105$), which is more or less acceptable. However, as discussed in Sect. 1.40, the sum of PaO_2 and $PaCO_2$ on room air should be about 140: in this case it is 120 (27 + 93). The defect in gas exchange can be better appreciated with the calculation of the A-aDO$_2$ (see also Sect. 1.42): **$PAO2 = FiO_2 (Pb - Pw) - PaCO_2/R$** Assuming a barometric pressure of 760 mmHg (sea level), and a respiratory quotient of 0.8: $PAO_2 = [0.21(760 - 47)] - (27/0.8) = 116$ $PAO_2-PaO_2 = 116 - 93 = 23$ A-aDO$_2$ = 23 (normally 7 – 14 on room air): **The A-aDO$_2$ is widened.**
0.1	*Acute respiratory acidosis*: not relevant
0.2	**Acute respiratory alkalosis:** $\Delta HCO_3^- = \Delta CO_2 \times 0.2$ $\Delta HCO_3^- = (40 - 27) \times 0.2 = 2.6$ Expected $HCO_3^- = 24 - 2.6 = 21.4$ Actual HCO_3^- (22) is almost identical with the expected HCO_3^- (21.4). The anion gap is also stated to be normal. **No associated metabolic disorder is present**
0.4	*Chronic respiratory acidosis:* not relevant
0.5	*Chronic respiratory alkalosis:* not relevant

Clinical correlation:
***Oxygenation: There seems to be a potential problem. In the absence of gross clinical and radiological abnormalities, pulmonary embolism should be considered even though the PaO_2 (93 mmHg) is roughly normal.

Normal $PaCO_2 = 40$ mmHg; Normal $HCO_3 = 24$ mEq/L; $\Delta =$ change in

13

13.12   Patient L: A 22 year-old man with a Head Injury

A 22 year old man was brought to the ER after suffering a head injury.

pH 7.58 PaCO$_2$: 27 mmHg HCO$_3^-$: 22 mEq/L. The anion gap is normal. PaO$_2$ 490 mmHg on FIO$_2$ 1.0.

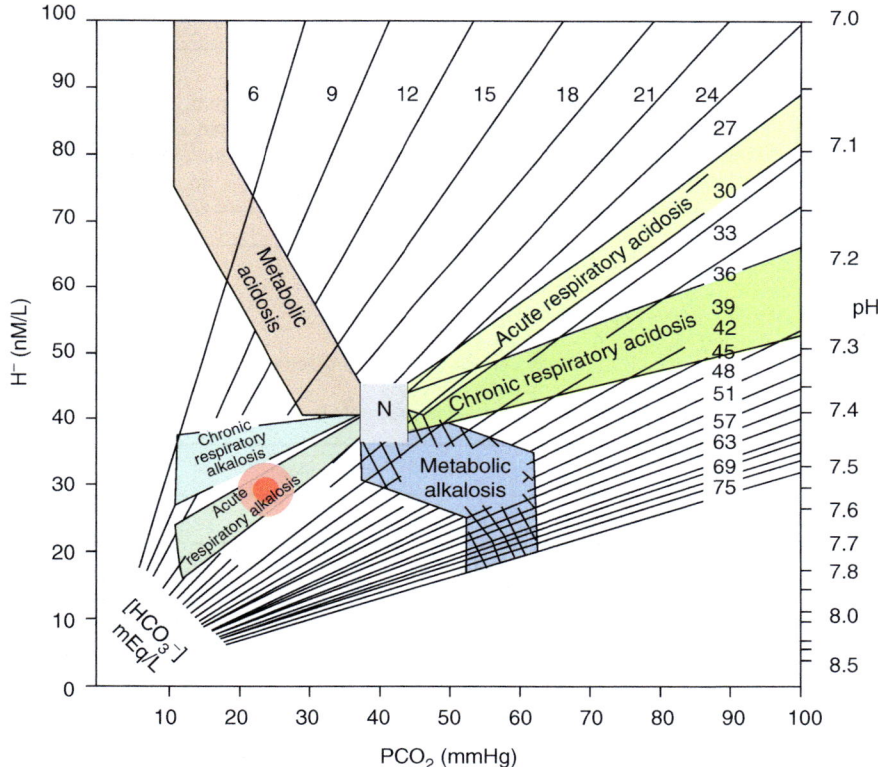

Patient L

As in the preceding example, this patient's values fall squarely on the band that represents acute respiratory alkalosis. A simple acid-base disorder, acute respiratory alkalosis, is present.

13

pH 7.58: Alkalemic	
Is metabolic alkalosis present (is the bicarbonate high?)	Is respiratory alkalosis present (is the $PaCO_2$ low?)
No	Yes. Is an associated metabolic disorder present? Apply the formula for *Acute Respiratory Alkalosis*. (Note that the anion gapis normal: there is no metabolic acidosis)

THE RESPIRATORY TRACK: 0-1-2-(3)-4-5

O	*Oxygenation:*
	The PaO_2 is 490 mmHg on FIO_2 of 1.0, which is virtually normal. Therefore, normal gas exchange mechanisms within the lung are anticipated, and there is unlikely to be any underlying lung injury eg, contusion, pneumothorax or a large hemothorax
0.1	*Acute respiratory acidosis:* Not relevant in this case.
0.2	Acute respiratory alkalosis: $\Delta HCO_3 = \Delta CO_2 \times 0.2$ $\Delta HCO_3 = (40 - 27) \times 0.2 = 2.6$ Expected $HCO_3 = 24 - 2.6 = 21.4$ The measured HCO_3 (22) is very close to that predicted (21.4). The anion gap is also normal. **No associated metabolic disorder is present**
0.4	*Chronic respiratory acidosis:* Not relevant in this case.
0.5	*Chronic respiratory alkalosis:* Not relevant in this case.

Clinical correlation:
The respiratory alkalosis is secondary to the hyperventilation consequent upon the cerebral injury. The gas oxygenation is normal: the lungs appear to be unaffected (there is no evidence of pulmonary contusion or neurogenic pulmonary edema).

13

13.13   Patient M: A 72 year-old man with Bronchopneumonia

A 72 year old man with COPD is brought to the ER with bronchopneumonia. He is
hypotensive and oliguric.

pH: 7.01, HCO_3: 24 mEq/L, PCO_2: 100 mmHg, PO_2: 40 mmHg on room air.

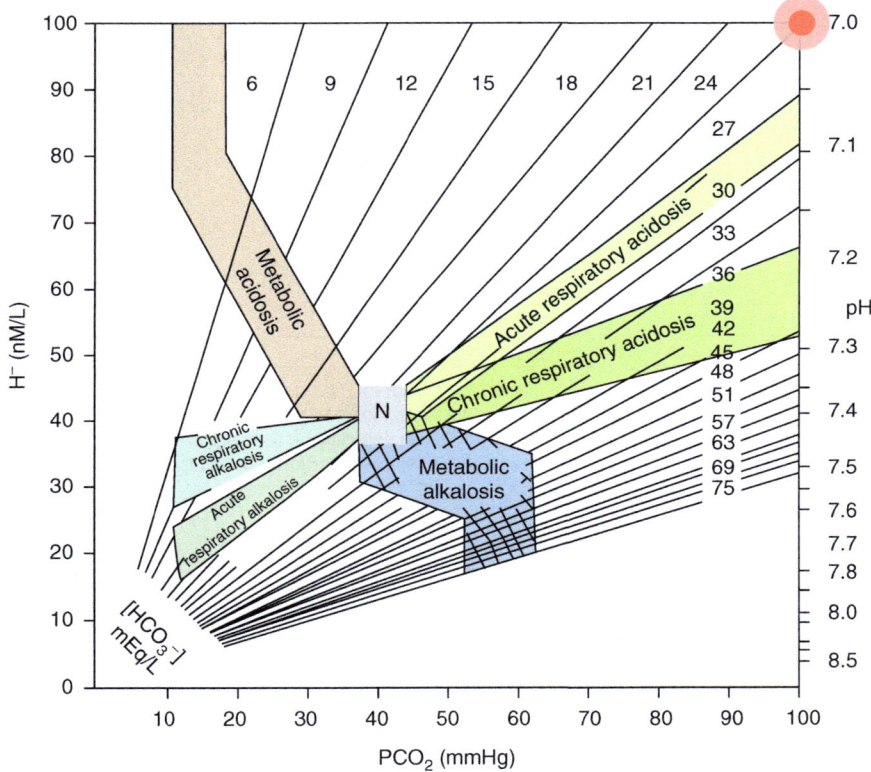

Patient M

This patients values have been graphed between the bands representing acute respiratory acidosis and metabolic acidosis, both of which can be shown to be present
(see algorithm opposite).

13

pH Acidemic	
Is it a *metabolic acidosis* that is the primary disorder, i.e., is the bicarbonate decreased? No, not (at first sight), at least	Is it a *respiratory acidosis* that is the primary disorder, i.e., is the CO_2 high? Yes. A primary respiratory acidosis is present.Go to *Respiratory Track*: apply the formula for *Acute Respiratory Acidosis:*

THE RESPIRATORY TRACK: 0-1-2-(3)-4-5	
O	*Oxygenation, assessment of:* The PaO_2 is 40 mmHg on 21 % O_2. With normal lungs the PaO_2 on 50 % O_2 would be expected to be roughly $21 \times 5 = 105$. In this case the PaO_2 (40 mmHg) is very low. The patient is severely hypoxemic.
0.1	**Is an associated metabolic disorder present?** Expected $HCO_3 = 24 + [(CO_2 - 40) \times 0.1]$ Expected $HCO_3 = 24 + [(100 - 40) \times 0.1]$ Expected $HCO_3 = 30$ The measured HCO_3 (24) is lower than the predicted HCO_3 (30). There appears to be a slight primary metabolic acidosis as well.
0.2	*Acute respiratory alkalosis:* Not relevant here.
0.4	*Chronic respiratory acidosis:* Not relevant here.
0.5	*Chronic respiratory alkalosis:* Not relevant here.
A	A metabolic acidosis is suspected (see above). *The anion gap is widened.* An associated wide-anion gap metabolic acidosis is present. In view of the severe hypoxemia (see next column), a lactic acidosis consequent upon reduced tissue perfusion is possible.Consider measuring serum lactate

Clinical Correlation
The clinical picture is consistent with the acute respiratory acidosis of a COPD exacerbation. Lactic acidosis due to poor organ perfusion and sepsis are likely responsible for the metabolic acidosis. Acute oliguric renal failure may also be incipient.
The associated hypoxemia is consistent with the pneumonia

13

13.14   Patient N: A 70 year-old woman with a Cerebrovascular Event

A 70 year old woman is brought to the ER with a cerebrovascular event.

pH: 7.10, HCO$_3^-$: 27 mEq/L, PCO$_2$: 88 mmHg, PO$_2$: 220 mmHg (on 50 % oxygen by Venturi-mask). The anion gap is normal.

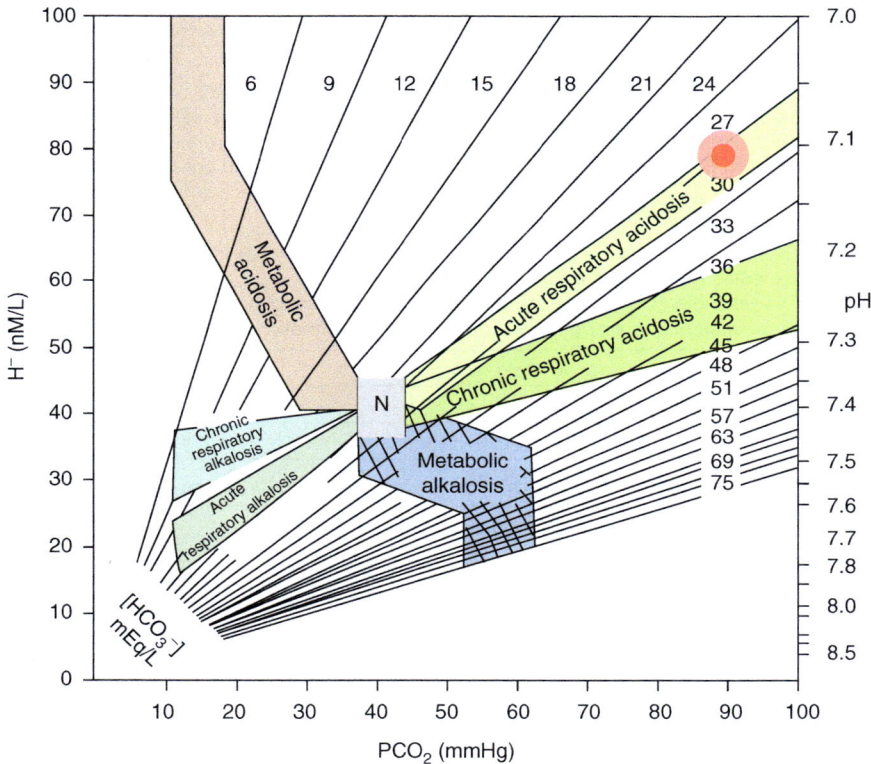

Patient N

This patient's values fall on the band representing acute respiratory acidosis. No associated acid-base disorder appears to be present.

13

pH: Acidemic	
Is metabolic acidosis the cause of the acidemia (is the bicarbonate low?)	Is respiratory acidosis the cause of the acidemia (is the PaCO$_2$ low?)
No	Yes. Is an associated metabolic disorder present? Apply the formula for *Acute Respiratory Alkalosis*.

THE RESPIRATORY TRACK: 0-1-2-(3)-4-5

O	*Oxygenation, assessment of:* The PaO$_2$ is 220 mmHg on 50 % O$_2$. With normal lungs the PaO$_2$ on 50 % O$_2$ would be expected to be roughly $50 \times 5 = 250$ (see 1.40). In this case the PaO$_2$ (220 mmHg) is very close to the expected PaO$_2$ for an FIO$_2$ of 0.5. Therefore a significant intrapulmonary oxygenating defect is virtually ruled out.
0.1	*Acute respiratory acidosis*: $\Delta HCO_3^- = \Delta CO_2 \times 0.1$ Expected HCO$_3$ = 24 + ΔHCO$_3^-$ Expected HCO$_3$ = 24 + [(CO$_2$ − 40) × 0.1] or, 24 + [(88 − 40) × 0.1] Expected HCO$_3$= 28.8 mEq/L. The measured HCO$_3$ is 27 mEq/L, which is very close to the predicted value. *No associated metabolic disorder is present.* For confirmation check the anion gap.
0.2	*Acute respiratory alkalosis:* Not relevant
0.4	*Chronic respiratory acidosis:* Not relevant
0.5	*Chronic respiratory alkalosis:* Not relevant

Metabolic Track: The Anion Gap is also normal: No metabolic acidosis exists.

Clinical Correlation

The clinical picture is consistent with hypoventilation due to the neurologic injury.

13

13.15   Patient O: A 60 year-old man with COPD and Cor Pulmonale

A 60 year old man with COPD and cor pulmonale undergoing evaluation at the outpatient clinic has the following arterial blood gases: pH: 7.30, HCO$_3$: 33 mEq/L, PCO$_2$: 64 mmHg, PO$_2$: 50 mmHg on room air. The anion gap is normal.

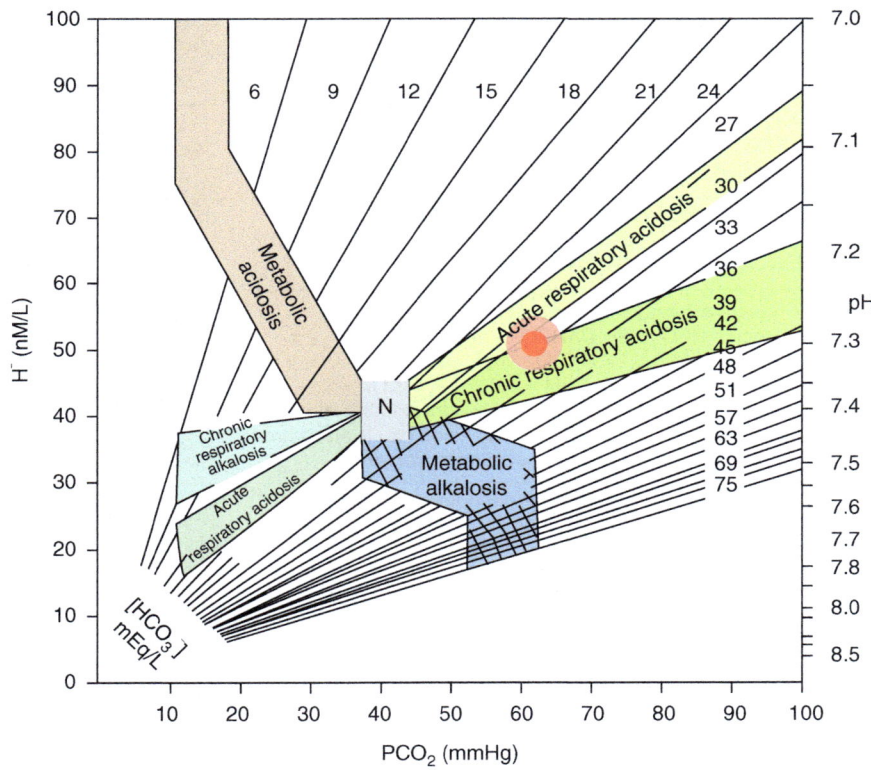

Patient O

Chronic respiratory acidosis.

pH is slightly on the acidemic side	
Is metabolic acidosis the cause of the acidemia (is the bicarbonate low?)	Is respiratory acidosis the cause of the acidemia (is the PaCO$_2$ high?)
No	Yes. A dominant respiratory acidosis is presents an associated metabolic disorder present? Apply the formula for *Chronic Respiratory Acidosis*

THE RESPIRATORY TRACK: 0-1-2-(3)-4-5	
O	*Oxygenation, assessment of:* Hypoxemia is present. This is Type 2 respiratory failure (the hypoxemia is associated with a raised PaCO$_2$).
0.1	*Acute respiratory acidosis:* (not relevant in this example) $\Delta HCO_3 = \Delta CO_2 \times 0.1$ Expected $HCO_3 = 24 + \Delta HCO_3$
0.2	*Acute respiratory alkalosis:* (not relevant in this example) $\Delta HCO_3 = \Delta CO_2 \times 0.2$ Expected $HCO_3 = 24 - \Delta HCO_3$
0.4	*Chronic respiratory acidosis:* $\Delta HCO_3 = \Delta CO_2 \times 0.4$ Expected $HCO_3 = 24 + \Delta HCO_3$ Expected $HCO_3 = 24 + [(CO_2 - 40) \times 0.4]$ Expected $HCO_3 = 24 + [(64 - 40) \times 0.4] = 33.6$ The measured HCO_3 (33 mEq/L) is almost identical to the expected HCO_3 (33.6 mEq/L). The anion gap is also normal. **No associated metabolic disorder is present.**
0.5	*Chronic respiratory alkalosis:* (not relevant in this example) $\Delta HCO_3 = \Delta CO_2 \times 0.5$ Expected $HCO_3 = 24 - \Delta HCO_3$
Clinical Correlation:	
The clinical picture is consistent with the chronic hypoventilation (Type 2 respiratory failure) of COPD.	

13

13.16   Patient P: A 70 year-old smoker with Acute Exacerbation of Chronic Bronchitis

A 70 year old smoker is admitted with "acute" exacerbation of chronic bronchitis. pH: 7.20, HCO_3^-: 24 mEq/l, PCO_2: 63 mmHg, PO_2: 52 mmHg on room air.

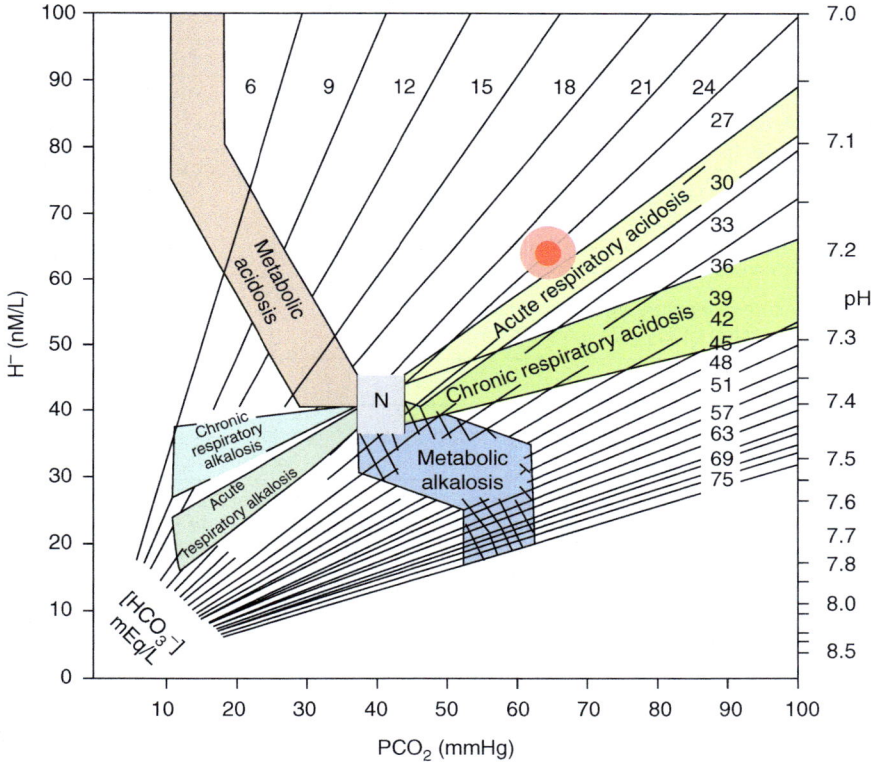

Patient P

The point plotted on this graph is close to the band for respiratory acidosis—in fact it lies between this band and the band of metabolic acidosis. As the algorithm on the opposite page suggests, both respiratory acidosis and metabolic acidosis are present.

13

pH: Acidemic	
Is metabolic acidosis the cause of the acidemia (is the bicarbonate low?)	Is respiratory acidosis the cause of the acidemia (is the $PaCO_2$ high?)
No.	Yes. A dominant respiratory acidosis is present. Is an associated metabolic disorder present? Apply the formula for *Chronic Respiratory Alkalosis*.

THE RESPIRATORY TRACK: 0-1-2-3-4-5

O	*Oxygenation, assessment of:* PaO_2 (52 mmHg) is low.
0.1	*Acute respiratory acidosis:* $\Delta HCO_3^- = \Delta CO_2 \times 0.1$ Expected $HCO_3 = 24 + \Delta HCO_3^-$ Expected $HCO_3^- = 24 + [(CO_2 - 40) \times 0.1]$ Expected $HCO_3^- = 24 + [(63 - 40) \times 0.1] = 24.3$ The measured HCO_3^- (24) is about the same (24.3 mEq/L). No gross metabolic process is apparent.
0.2	*Acute respiratory alkalosis:* $\Delta HCO_3^- = \Delta CO_2 \times 0.2$ Expected $HCO_3 = 24 - \Delta HCO_3^-$
0.4	*Chronic respiratory acidosis:* $\Delta HCO_3 = \Delta CO_2 \times 0.4$
0.5	*Chronic respiratory alkalosis:* $\Delta HCO_3^- = \Delta CO_2 \times 0.5$ Expected $HCO_3^- = 24 - \Delta HCO_3^-$

This is the classical acute exacerbation in COPD. Care must be taken to give the *minimum possible* FIO_2 to achieve an acceptable PaO_2 (of about 60 mmHg). This is to avoid inadvertent suppression of the respiratory drive. The associated metabolic acidosis could be lactic (PaO_2 is low), but must be worked up in its own merits.

13

13.17   Patient Q: A 50 year-old man with Hematemesis

A 55 year old man is admitted with severe hematemesis. His hemoglobin is found to be 4.5 g/dL.

   pH: 7.35, $PaCO_2$: 34 mmHg, HCO_3: 18 mEq/L, PaO_2: 89 mmHg and SpO_2: 97 % on room air. His anion gap is elevated.

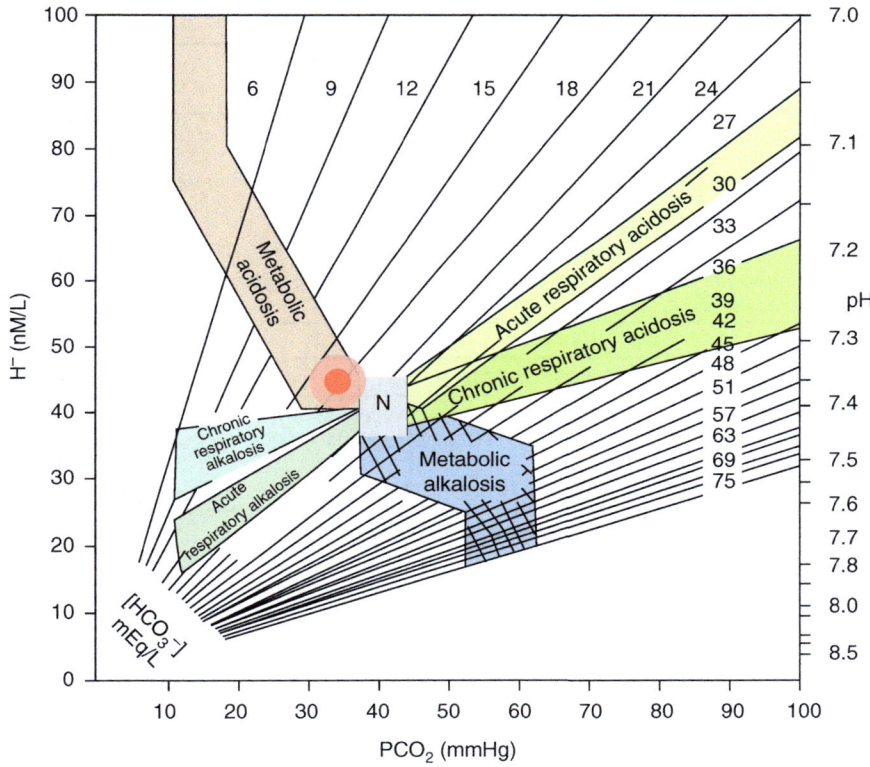

Patient Q

Metabolic acidosis

pH 7.35: Slightly acidemic	
Is metabolic acidosis the cause of the acidemia (is the bicarbonate low?)	Is respiratory acidosis the cause of the acidemia (is the $PaCO_2$ high?)
Yes. A dominant metabolic acidosis is present	No

THE METABOLIC TRACK: A-B-C-D-E	
A	*Anion gap*: high (See ***D*** below)
B	*Bicarbonate gap: $\Delta AG - \Delta HCO_3$ (Should be calculated. See examples further on)*
C	*Colloid gap: Measured osmolality minus calculated osmolarlity. Should be assessed in the relevant situation*
D	*Disorder, associated primary respiratory: The acidosis is a wide anion gap metabolic acidosis.* Is an associated respiratory disorder present? *Apply Winter's formula:* Predicted $CO_2 = (1.5 \times HCO_3) + 8\pm2$ Predicted $CO_2 = (1.5 \times 18) + 8\pm2 = 35$ mmHg Actual CO_2 (34) falls within the predicted range (33–37). *There is full respiratory compensation for the metabolic acidosis. No associated primary respiratory disorder is present.*
E	*Electrolytes, urinary: UAG $= [Na^+] + [K^+] - [Cl^-]$*

RESPIRATORY TRACK: OXYGENATION	
O	How is the fall in hemoglobin impacting on oxygen delivery? $CaO_2 = 1.34 \times Hb \times SpO_2$ (see 00.00 Sect. 1.22 and 1.23) $CaO_2 = 1.34 \times 4.5 \times 97$ $CaO_2 = 5.7$ mL O_2/dL (normal $=16$–22 mL O_2/dL)

Clinical Correlation:
The oxygen delivery is reduced to about a third of normal. This is capable of causing tissue hypoperfusion and lactic acidosis, which could be the cause of the wide anion gap metabolic acidosis.

13

13.18   Patient R: A 68 year-old man with an Acute Abdomen

A 68 year old man has been diagnosed with an acute abdomen. He has been vomiting for the last few days, and is dehydrated.

pH: 7.50 HCO_3: 36 mEq/L, $PaCO_2$: 44 mmHg. Na^+: 134 mEq/L, K^+: 2.7 mEq/L, Cl^-: 90 mEq/L, Urinary spot chloride: <10 mEq/L.

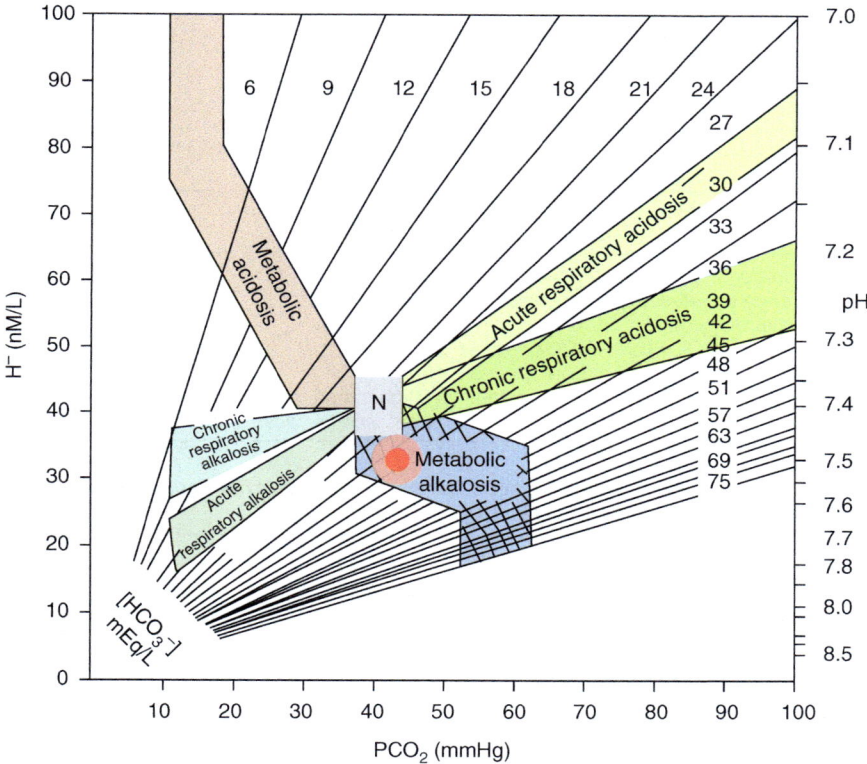

Patient R

Metabolic alkalosis. Based on acid-base mapping alone, no other acid-base disturbance is expected to coexist. However the method is not infallible, and as the discussion on the facing page shows, an associated respiratory acidosis is in fact present.

13

pH 7.58; Alkalemic	
Is metabolic alkalosis the cause of the alkalosis (is the bicarbonate high?)	Is respiratory alkalosis the cause of the alkalosis (is the PaCO$_2$ low?)
Yes. A dominant metabolic alkalosis is present	No

THE METABOLIC TRACK: A-B-C-D-E	
A	Anion gap. **Is an associated metabolic disorder present?** Calculate the anion gap (AG): AG = Na$^+$ – (Cl$^-$ + HCO$_3$) AG = 134 – (90 + 36) = 8 The AG is normal. There is no associated metabolic acidosis.
B	Bicarbonate gap: $\Delta AG - \Delta HCO_3$. Not relevant since no associated metabolic acidosis is present.
C	Colloid gap: Measured osmolality minus calculated osmolarlity. Not relevant since no associated metabolic acidosis is present.
D	Disorder, associated primary respiratory: Is an associated respiratory disorder present? Actual CO$_2$ = 44.6 Predicted CO$_2$ = (0.7 × HCO$_3$) + 21+/–5 Predicted CO$_2$ = (0.7 × 36) + 21+/–5 = 46.2 Actual CO$_2$ (46.2 mmHg) is substantially higher than predicted 36 An associated respiratory acidosis is present, and its cause should be sought.
E	Electrolytes, urinary: Characterize the metabolic alkalosis: is it chloride-resistant or chloride-responsive? The urinary spot chloride is low (<10).

Clinical Correlation
The urinary chloride is low, consistent with dehydration and also with the loss of chloride by vomiting. The hypochloremia and the hypokalemia, unless corrected, could perpetuate the metabolic alkalosis.

13

13.19   Patient S: A young woman with Gastroenteritis and Dehydration

A young woman is admitted with dehydration due to gastroenteritis.

pH: 7.39, PCO_2: 39 mmHg, HCO_3: 21 mEq/L, Na^+: 145 mEq/L, K^+: 3.2 mEq/L, Cl^-: 94 mEq/L

At first sight, the pH is normal, and there is no obvious acid-base abnormality.

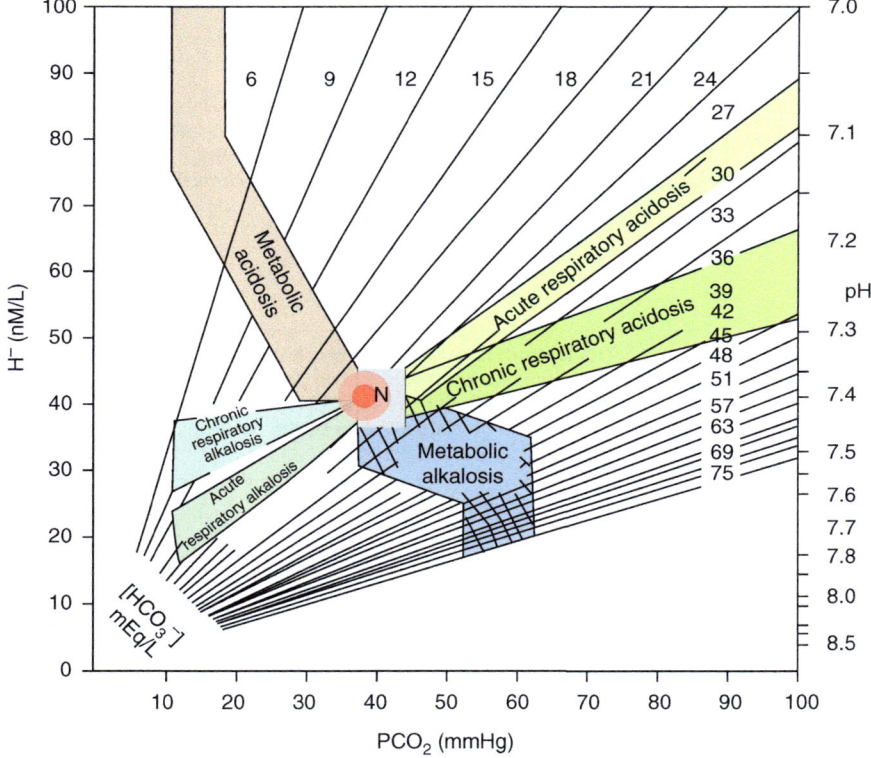

Patient S

The point plotted falls in the zone of normality, but this can occur when a metabolic acidosis is opposed by a metabolic alkalosis (see discussion on facing page).

13

Note that the anion gap is clearly widened:
$$AG = [Na^+] - ([Cl^-] - [HCO_3])$$
$$AG = 145 - (21 + 94)$$
$$AG = 30$$
There is a wide anion gap metabolic acidosis

Is an associated metabolic alkalosis present?
Calculate the Delta Ratio = $\Delta AG - \Delta HCO_3$
$= (30 - 12) - (24 - 21) = 15$ (normal +6 to –6)
(Recall that if the Delta Ratio is > +6 mEq/L, an associated
metabolic alkalosis is present , if < +6 mEq/L, an associated
narrow-anion gap metabolic acidosis is present).
*There is a coexistent metabolic alkalosis that is "neutralizing"
the metabolic acidosis.*

The Bottom line: Clinical Correlation
The metabolic acidosis is presumably on account of the
hypoperfusion and a possible pre-renal component. The
metabolic alkalosis can be accounted for by the dehydration
and volume contraction.

13

13.20   Patient T: A 50 year-old woman with Paralytic Ileus

A 50 year old woman with post-operative paralytic ileus has the following blood gases:

pH: 7.58, HCO₃: 50 mEq/L, PCO₂: 52 mmHg. The anion gap is normal.

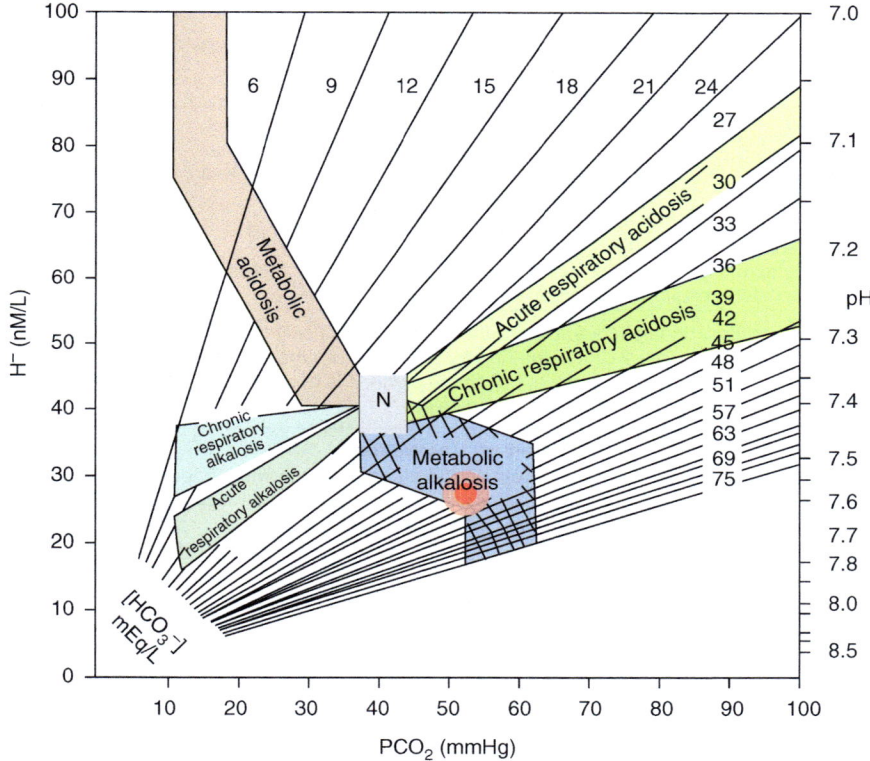

Patient T

One of the limitations of the acid-base mapping is that it is not possible to diagnose a "triple disorder" by this method. Although the above patient's values fall well within the band of metabolic alkalosis, there are two additional coexistent acid-base disturbances, as the algorithm on the opposite page reveals.

13

pH 7.58: Alkalemic	
Is metabolic alkalosis the cause of the alkalemia (is the bicarbonate high?)	Is respiratory acidosis the cause of the alkalemia (is the PaCO$_2$ low?)
Yes	No

	THE METABOLIC TRACK: A-B-C-D-E
A	*Anion gap. Is another metabolic disorder (viz, metabolic acidosis) also present?* *Calculate the anion gap* (AG): AG = Na$^+$ − (Cl$^-$ + HCO$_3^-$) However, the anion gap has been stated to be normal. There is no metabolic acidosis.
B	*Bicarbonate gap: $\Delta AG - \Delta HCO_3$*
C	*Colloid gap: Measured osmolality minus calculated osmolarlity*
D	*Disorder, associated primary respiratory. Use the equation relevant to metabolic alkalosis:* Predicted PCO$_2$ = (0.7 × HCO$_3^-$) + 21±5 Predicted CO$_2$ = (50 × 0.7) + 21±5 = 56±5 The actual CO$_2$ (52) falls within the expected range (51 − 61) so there is no apparent coexistent respiratory disorder
E	*Electrolytes, urinary: Characterize the metabolic alkalosis: is it chloride-resistant or chloride-responsive?* Check the urinary spot chloride (the urinary spot sodium has not been done in this example, but all the same, it is necessary for the further characterization of the metabolic alkalosis).

Clinical Correlation
Metabolic alkalosis, for a variety of reasons, is a common accompaniment of paralytic ileus.

13

13.21   Patient U: An 80 year-old woman with Extreme Weakness

An 89 year old woman on diuretic therapy presented to the ER with extreme weakness. pH: 7.55, PCO$_2$: 50 mmHg, HCO$_3^-$: 44.4 mEq/L, Na$^+$: 144 mEq/L, K$^+$: 2.0 mEq/L, Cl$^-$: 90 mEq/L; Urinary Spot Chloride: 72 mEq/L

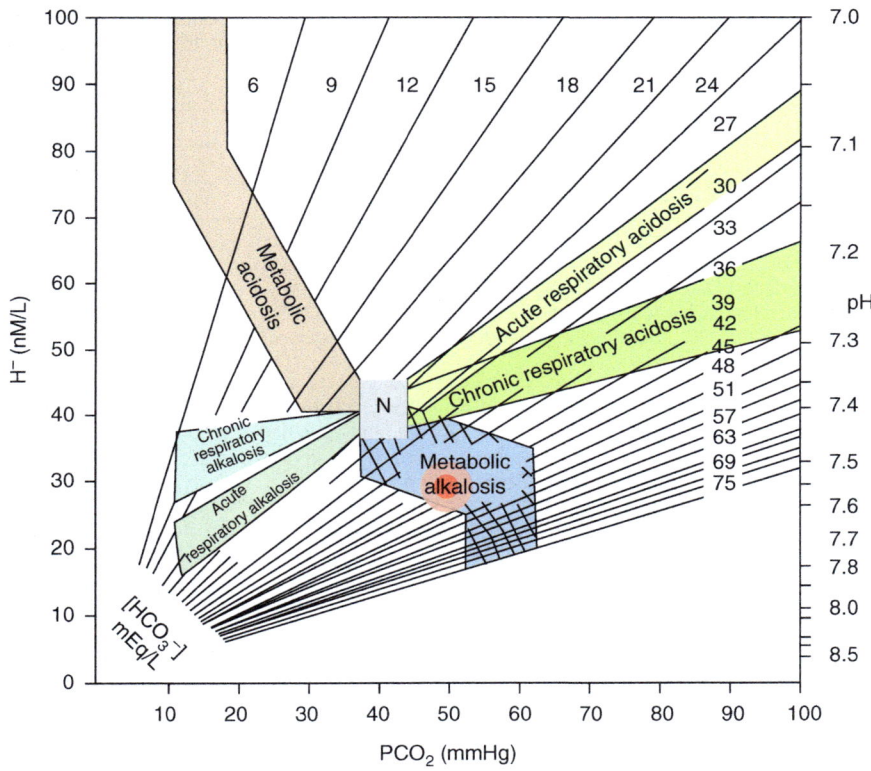

Patient U

Metabolic alkalosis

13

pH 7.55: **alkalemic**	
Is metabolic alkalosis the cause of the acidemia (is the bicarbonate high?)	Is respiratory acidosis the cause of the acidemia (is the PaCO$_2$ high?)
Yes. A dominant metabolic alkalosis is present. Go to the METABOLIC TRACK	No
THE METABOLIC TRACK: A-B-C-D-E	

A	*Anion gap. Is an associated metabolic disorder present?* There is no reason to suspect a metabolic acidosis in this case, but sometimes metabolic acidosis and metabolic alkalosis can coexist. Calculate the anion gap AG = Na$^+$ − (Cl$^-$ = HCO$_3^-$) = 144 − (90 + 50) = 4. No metabolic acidosis coexists.
B	*Bicarbonate gap: ΔAG − ΔHCO$_3^-$: Not relevant in this case.*
C	*Colloid gap: Measured osmolality minus calculated osmolarlity. Not relevant in this case.*
D	*Disorder, associated primary respiratory: Is an associated respiratory disorder present?* Predicted CO$_2$ = [(0.7 × HCO$_3^-$) + 21] ±5 Predicted CO$_2$ = [(0.7 × 44.4) + 21] ±5 = 52±5 = 47–57 The actual CO$_2$ (50 mmHg) is within this range. *No associated respiratory disorder is present.*
E	*Electrolytes, urinary: Characterize the metabolic alkalosis: is it chloride-resistant or chloride-responsive?* The urinary spot chloride 72 is high (i.e., >40 mEq/L). This can be associated with severe hypokalemia, current usage of diuretics or with mineralocorticoid excess (Sects. 10.2 and 10.11).
Clinical correlation:	
The inciting mechanism for the metabolic alkalosis is likely the diuretic usage. The predominant maintenance factor appears to be the severe hypokalemia.	

13

13.22   Patient V: A 50 year-old man with Diarrhea

A 50 year old man presents to the ER with severe diarrhea since 4 days. He is dehydrated.

pH: 7.18 HCO$_3^-$: 6.0 mEq/L, PCO$_2$: 19 mmHg, Na$^+$: 130 mEq/L, K$^+$: 2.6 mEq/L, Cl$^-$: 114 mEq/L

pH 7.18: **acidemic**

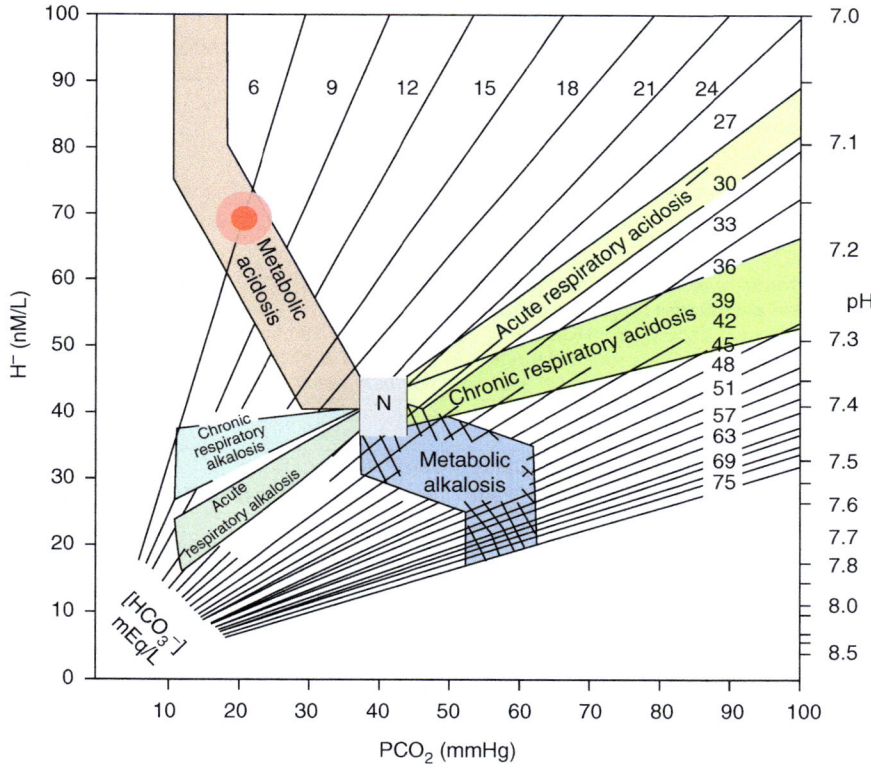

Patient V

Metabolic acidosis

pH 7.18: **acidemic**	
Is it a *metabolic acidosis* that is the dominant disorder, i.e., is the bicarbonate low?	Is it a *respiratory acidosis* that is dominant, i.e., is the CO_2 high?
Yes. A dominant metabolic acidosis is present. Go to the METABOLIC TRACK	No

THE METABOLIC TRACK: A-B-C-D-E	
A	*Anion gap. Is an associated metabolic disorder present?* AG = $[Na^+] - (Cl^- + HCO_3^-) = 130 - (114 + 6) = 10$. The anion gap is normal. *The acidosis is a normal anion gap metabolic acidosis.*
B	*Bicarbonate gap (BG): $\Delta AG - \Delta HCO_3^-$:* **Is an associated metabolic disorder present?** BG = $\Delta AG - \Delta HCO_3^-$ = (approx zero) − (24−6). The BG is clearly negative (a BG more negative than −6: supports the diagnosis of a hyperchloremic metabolic acidosis).
C	*Colloid gap: Not relevant in this case.*
D	*Disorder, associated primary respiratory:* **Is an associated respiratory disorder present?** Predicted CO_2 = $[(1.5 \times HCO_3) + 8] \pm 2 = 17\pm2 = 15$–19 mmHg The actual CO_2 (19) falls within the predicted range (15–19). There is full respiratory compensation for the metabolic acidosis. *No associated primary respiratory disorder is present.*
E	*Electrolytes, urinary: Characterize the metabolic alkalosis in the relevant situation.*

| **Clinical Correlation** |
| The commonest cause of a hyperchloremic metabolic acidosis is diarrhea. |

13

13.23   Patient W: A 68 year-old woman with Congestive Cardiac Failure

A 68 year old female presented to the ER in severe congestive cardiac failure.
    pH: 7.62, HCO$_3^-$: 21 mEq/L, PCO$_2$: 25 mmHg, PaO$_2$ 65 mmHg on 50 % O$_2$ by
Venturi-mask. Na$^+$: 130 mEq/L, Cl$^-$: 80 mEq/L.

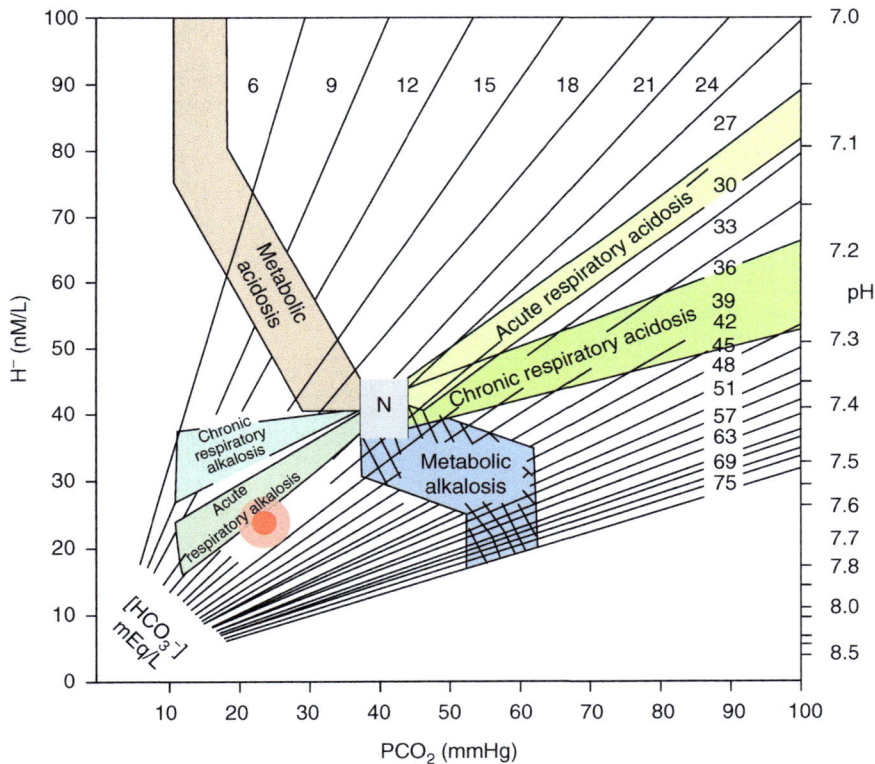

Patient W

To all appearances, an acute respiratory alkalosis with a probable metabolic alkalosis is present. As in the case of patient T, this patient's acid-base mapping has failed
to reveal a triple disorder(see discussion opposite).

13

pH: alkalemic	
Is metabolic acidosis the cause of the acidemia (is the bicarbonate high?)	Is respiratory acidosis the cause of the acidemia (is the $PaCO_2$ low?)
No: (but see below)	Yes: Go to the RESPIRATORY TRACK (0-1-2-3-4-5). *Is an associated metabolic disorder present?* Since the problem is several days old, apply the formula for *chronic respiratory acidosis.*
A *Anion gap: Even though no associated metabolic disorder appears to be present, check the anion gap anyway.* $AG = Na^+ - (Cl^- + HCO_3^-) = AG = 29$ A 'WAGMA' seems to be coexistent, though it was not anticipated initially. A metabolic alkalosis may be masking the acidosis, and the bicarbonate gap must now be checked.	**O** *Oxygenation, assessment of:* The PaO_2 is 65 mmHg on an FIO_2 of 0.5, which is low. (Predicted O_2 = approx $50\% \times 5 = 250$ mmHg: See Sect. 1.40).
B *Bicarbonate gap: $\Delta AG - \Delta HCO_3^-$* $= (27-12) - (24-21) = 12$ (i.e., >6mEq/L) An associated metabolic alkalosis is present.	**1** *Acute respiratory acidosis:*
C *Colloid gap:*	**2** *Acute respiratory alkalosis:*
D *Disorder, associated primary respiratory:*	**4** *Acute respiratory alkalosis:* Expected $HCO_3^- = 24 - [(40 - CO_2) \times 0.2] = 21$ (This identical to the measured HCO_3. *No associated metabolic disorder is apparent. However see anion gap and bicarbonate gap (top left).*
E *Electrolytes, urinary:*	**5** *Chronic respiratory alkalosis:*
Clinical correlation:	
All causes of a wide anion gap metabolic acidosis (Sect. 9.8) must be investigated. The *Bicarbonate gap* is wide as well. The patient has been vomiting, and on account of this, the third disorder—a coexistent met alkalosis-has supervened. The hypoxemia is likely on account of the congestive cardiac failure and pulmonary edema.	

13

13.24   Patient X: An 82 year-old woman with Diabetic Ketoacidosis

A 82 year old woman was admitted in diabetic ketoacidosis; she had been coughing and breathless for a few days, and a right lower lobe pneumonia was found at admission.

pH: 7.35, PCO_2: 25 mmHg, HCO_3^-: 18 mEq/L, Na^+: 141 mEq/L, Cl^-: 89 mEq/L, PaO_2 82 mmHg on 50 % O_2,

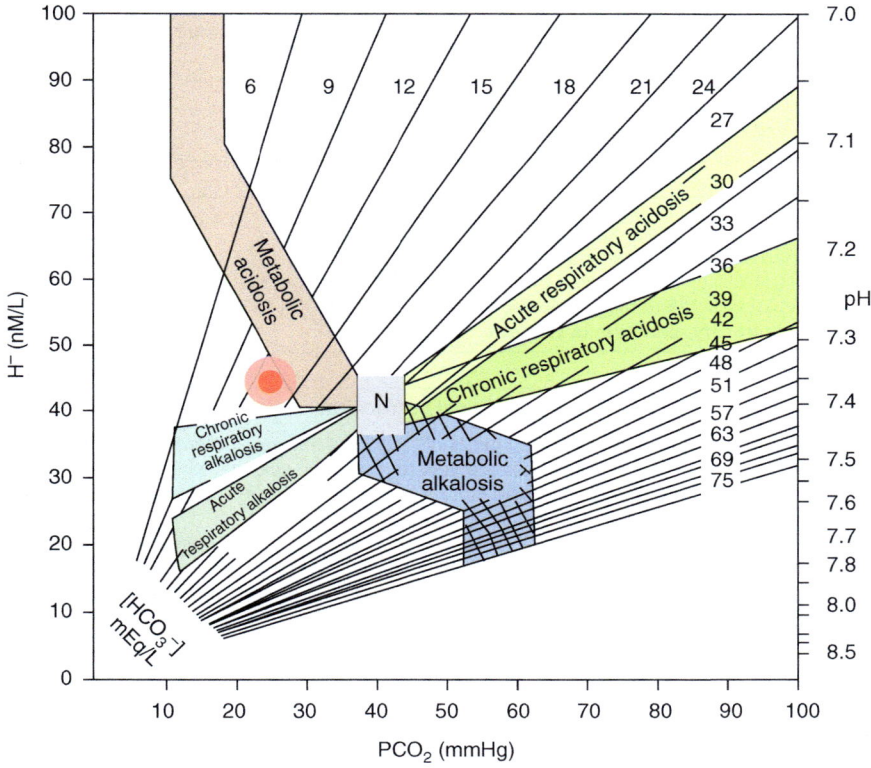

Patient X

Impression: metabolic acidosis with chronic respiratory alkalosis. In fact, a triple disorder is present (see discussion opposite).

13

	pH 7.36: mildly acidemic	
	Is metabolic acidosis present (is the bicarbonate low?)	Is respiratory acidosis present (is the PaCO$_2$ high?)
	Yes, marginally. A dominant metabolic acidosis is possibly present: Apply the METABOLIC TRACK	No
A	**Anion gap:** AG=[Na$^+$] − ([Cl$^-$] + [HCO$_3^-$]) = 141 − (89 + 18) = 34 The anion gap is widened. **The acidosis is a WAGMA**	
B	**Bicarbonate gap: Is an associated metabolic alkalosis present?** Calculate the bicarbonate gap (delta ratio) Delta ratio= ΔAG − ΔHCO$_3^-$ Delta ratio= (34 − 12) − (24 − 18)=16 (very high) **A coexisting metabolic alkalosis is present**	
C	*Colloid gap:*	
D	*Disorder, associated primary respiratory:* **Is an associated respiratory disorder present?** Actual CO$_2$ = 25 Predicted CO$_2$ = (1.5 × HCO3) + 8±2 = 35±2 mmHg Actual CO$_2$ (25 mmHg) is lower than the predicted CO$_2$ (33–37) **A primary respiratory alkalosis is present**	
E	*Electrolytes, urinary:*	
	Clinical correlation:	
	DKA presents with a wide anion gap metabolic acidosis. However there is a discrepancy: the substantially widened AG suggests a severe metabolic acidosis which is seemingly out of proportion to the mild depression in the serum bicarbonate.A coexisting metabolic alkalosis was suspected and confirmed (see also Sect. 9.36).	
	To explain the metabolic alkalosis, dyselectrolytemias (hypochloremia, hypokalemia) should be looked for, and a history of current diuretic therapy etc must be sought.	
	The respiratory alkalosis is consistent with the pneumonia.	

13

13.25   Patient Y: A 50 year-old male in Cardiac Arrest

A 50 year old male suffers a cardiopulmonary arrest in the ICU.

pH 7.0, HCO_3^-: 6.0 PCO_2: 29 mmHg, PaO_2 180 mmHg on FIO_2 100 % on ventilator. Na^+: 144 mEq/L, K^+: 5.0 mEq/L, Cl^-: 104 mEq/L.

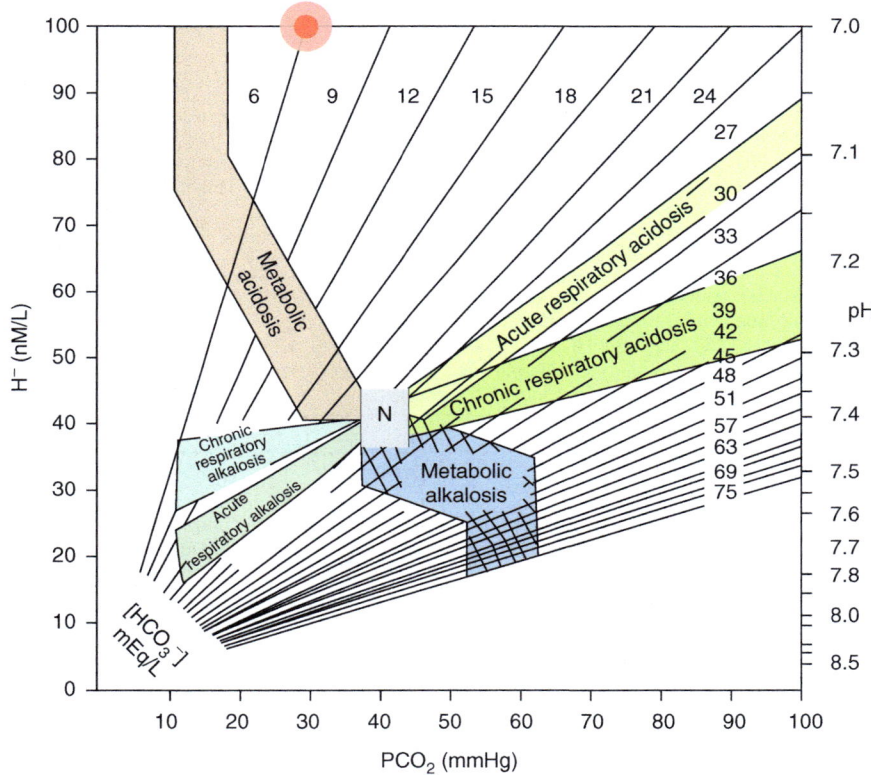

Patient Y
Severe metabolic acidosis with acute respiratory alkalosis.

13

pH 7.0: **Acidemic**	
Is it a metabolic acidosis that is the dominant disorder, i.e., is the bicarbonate low?	Is respiratory acidosis the cause of the acidemia (is the $PaCO_2$ high?)
Yes. A dominant metabolic acidosis is present.	No, not at first sight.

	THE METABOLIC TRACK: A-B-C-D-E
A	*Anion gap*. Characterize the metabolic acidosis. AG = $[Na^+]$ + ($[Cl^-]$ + $[HCO_3^-]$) = 144 − (104 + 6.0) = 32 The anion gap is widened. *The acidosis is a WAGMA.*
B	*Bicarbonate gap: $\Delta AG - \Delta HCO_3$.* *Is an associated metabolic alkalosis present?* Unlikely, but calculate the bicarbonate gap anyway. *BG = ($\Delta AG - \Delta HCO_3$) = (32 −12) − (24 − 6) = 2.* This falls within the normal range (−6 to +6). *No associated metabolic alkalosis.*
C	*Colloid gap: Measured osmolality minus calculated osmolarlity*
D	*Disorder, associated primary respiratory:* Is an associated respiratory disorder present? Predicted CO_2 = [(1.5 × HCO_3) + 8] ±2 = [(1.5 x 6) + 8] ±2 = 17±2. Actual CO_2 (29 mmHg) significantly exceeds the predicted CO_3 (15 − 19 mmHg). *A primary respiratory acidosis is also present.*
E	*Electrolytes, urinary.*
	Clinical correlation Lactic acidosis as a consequence of the CP arrest is the likely cause of the WAGMA. There may also now be an element of renal failure, and the creatinine needs to be checked as well. Cardiopulmonary arrest accounts for the respiratory acidosis (hypoventilation). A PaO_2 of 180 is lower than expected on a FIO_2 of 1.0. A chest x-ray must be obtained to rule out a pneumothorax (which can occur post-CPR), lobar atelectasis, aspiration pneumonia etc.

13

13.26   Patient Z: A 50 year-old Diabetic with Cellulitis

A 50 year old diabetic with chronic kidney disease is admitted with cellulitis of the leg. a deep venous thrombosis is also suspected. He has been breathless for less than a day. He is dehydrated but not in ketoacidosis.

pH: 7.45, $PaCO_2$: 25 mmHg, HCO_3^-: 15 mEq/L, Na^+: 144 mEq/L, Cl^-: 95 mEq/L, PaO_2: 55 mmHg on room air.

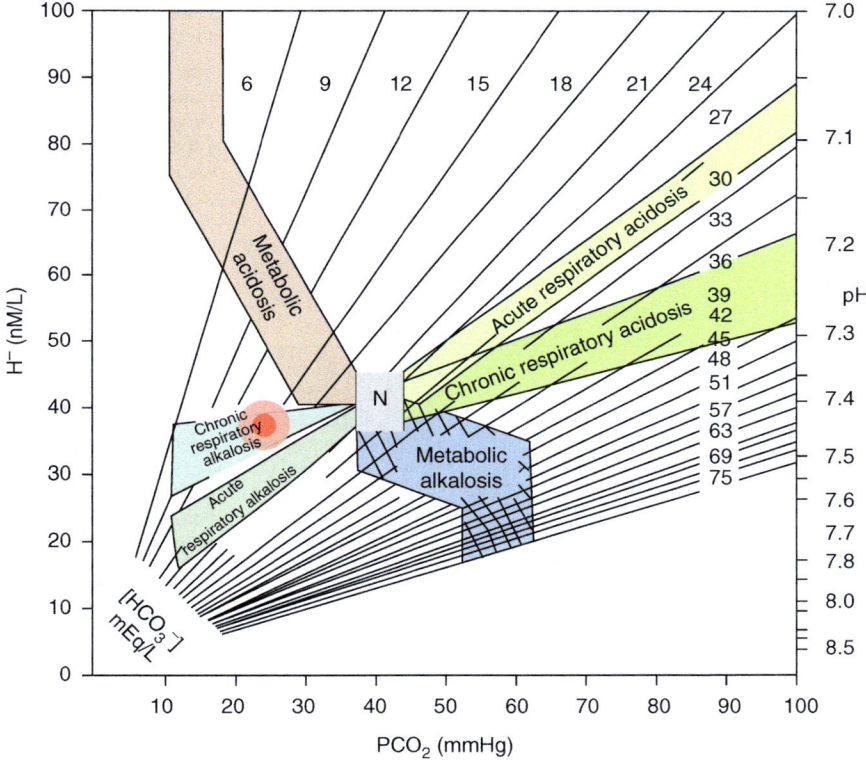

This patient's acid-base map conveys the impression of chronic respiratory alkalosis. In actual fact, a triple disorder is present (see discussion opposite).

13

pH: alkalemic		
Is metabolic acidosis the cause of the acidemia (is the bicarbonate high?)		Is respiratory acidosis the cause of the acidemia (is the $PaCO_2$ low?)
No		Yes. A dominant respiratory alkalosis is present. Go to the RESPIRATORY TRACK (0-1-2-3-4-5): *Is an associated metabolic disorder present?* Apply the formula for a cute respiratory alkalosis.
A	*Anion gap*: AG = $[Na^+] - ([Cl^-] + [HCO_3^-])$ AG = $144 - (95 + 15)$ AG = 34 *The acidosis is a wide anion gap metabolic acidosis. Calculate the bicarbonate gap (below).*	**O**	*Oxygenation, assessment of:* The PaO_2 is 55 mmHg on room air. This is low, more so since the patient is hyperventilating (as evidenced by the low $PaCO_2$).
B	*Bicarbonate gap*: $\Delta AG - \Delta HCO_3$ Delta ratio = $(34 - 12) - (24 - 15)$ Delta ratio = 13 *A metabolic alkalosis is also present.*	**1**	*Acute respiratory acidosis:* *Not relevant here.*
C	*Colloid gap*: Measured osmolality minus calculated osmolarlity Osmolarlity: $(2 \times Na)$ + glucose/18 + BUN/2.8 (Calculate the colloid gap in the appropriate clinical situation after ruling out DKA, lactic acidosis, uremia and salicylate poisoning which can also widen it).	**2**	*Acute respiratory alkalosis:* Expected HCO_3 = $(40 - CO_2)$ x 0.2± Expected HCO_3 = $24 - [(40 - 25)$ x $0.2]$ Expected HCO_3 = 21 Actual HCO_3 (15) is lower than expected (21). *There is an associated metabolic acidosis. Now check the anion gap.*
D	*Disorder, associated primary respiratory:* Not relevant here.	**4**	*Chronic respiratory acidosis:* *Not relevant here.*
E	*Electrolytes, urinary:* *Not relevant here.*	**5**	*Chronic respiratory alkalosis:* *Not relevant here.*
Clinical correlation:		
The metabolic acidosis may be on account of acute-on-chronic kidney disease and sepsis. A cause for the metabolic alkalosis is likely the volume contraction. With hypoxemia and respiratory alkalosis in the setting of deep venous thrombosis, pulmonary thromboembolism requires to be ruled out.		

13

Index

The manufacturer's authorised representative in the EU is Springer
Nature Customer Service Centre GmbH, Europaplatz 3, 69115 Heidelberg,
Germany. If you have any concerns regarding our products, please
contact ProductSafety@springernature.com

Printed and bound by CPI Group (UK) Ltd, Croydon, CR0 4YY
23/04/2026
02095602-0005